THE OPIOID ALTERNATIVE

The Opioid Alternative

Medical Meditation
For Surgery-For Pain-For Life

By Dr. Scott M. Fried

ISBNs:
979-8-9856111-0-6
979-8-9856111-1-3

AUDIO SESSIONS FOR YOU

*This Book Has Four Audios for you to listen and learn
Medical Meditation.
You may begin listening at any time or wait until the chapter
matches the session as you read.
Each session is designed to help you develop your own personal
healing program
I hope you enjoy these as much as I did when recording them.*

**Page 63
Audio #1 An Introduction to Medical Meditation
How to do your Medical Meditation**

**Page 84
Audio #2 Begin your Medical Meditation
The Quick In-Out**

**Page 116
Audio #3 A Healing Session
Healing Sand**

**Page 156
Audio #4 Medical Meditation for Surgery and Healing
A Relaxing, Repeating Session for Surgery, Comfort
and Healing**

*You should not use these techniques or listen to the audio portion of
the program while driving, working with machinery or when doing
any activity that requires concentration and attention.*

*Download your audios at www.docinthehouse.com by using the ISBN
number (found above the bar code) of this book.*

ACKNOWLEDGEMENTS

This book is dedicated to my family, whose support and love allow me the privilege of living a life dedicated to helping people heal and have happier lives.

Laura, my rock, foundation, love of my life and my mirror you are amazing, and clearly my better half - thank you for always partnering with me on our path to help the world heal themselves.

Josh, Ally and Hannah are my three spirits who balance me, support my "eccentric ways" and keep me focused on what is important in life. You three are my greatest gifts, having outshined me already in most every way.

Thanks to my dear friend and mentor, Dr. Bernie Siegel, who taught me to hug my patients. Our patients become friends as well as teachers and each are healers in their own right.

I hope the words in this book, as well as the audios, give back in a small way all the love and caring I have received from most everyone I have met in my career as well as personal life.

Life is to be lived, and if I can help a few people enjoy the experience of living, without blunting that joy with drugs, it will have been well worth writing.

Thank each of you for sharing this journey with me.

INTRODUCTION

The opioid crisis is real, and since the recent pandemic, this has reached even higher epidemic proportions! Many who lost their jobs or whose lives were otherwise disrupted turned to drugs or addictive medications to deal with their real-life stresses.

We tend to forget as well that chronic pain and sleep dysfunction, often accompanied by a sense of helplessness in caring for ourselves, are overwhelming issues that have devastated and destroyed many families and their loved ones.

This is what this book is about: facing these problems head-on—the everyday, real-life problems, not the crises that distract us from them.

This book is about answers—real solutions for you and those you love, to allow each of us to take control of our own lives and health so that we are not the next victims of a crisis, injury, or medical challenge.

I offer you real-world, simple, effective, and easy-to-use techniques to take control of your life so that each emergency situation and life challenge that's thrown at you doesn't send you into a downward health and life spiral and distract you from what is destined, if you envision it—a wonderful, happy, and healthy life! That's exactly what will manifest for anyone who wants it!

Let's begin this journey together.

CHAPTER 1

The statistics are staggering.

Millions become addicted to opioid painkillers, antidepressants, and mind-altering medications every year. Getting off these has become a nightmare for many who lived normal lives until a simple medical procedure or trial of a medication sent their lives into living hell. These challenges ruin lives, destroy minds and bodies, tear apart families, and devastate careers.

We have all been sold a bill of goods: "The medical community will take care of you!" The reality is that only one person can care for you best—and that is you. Being in control of your world, what you feel, and how you deal with pain, injury, and emotional or physical crises often defines your life path and in many cases who you are.

The opioid crisis is not limited to painkillers and narcotic medications; it extends to all aspects of medical care.

The medical literature shows that the antidepressants used for everything from pain management and depression to ADD, as well as a plethora of medication choices for the problem du jour—pills for sleep disorders, muscle relaxers for spasms, antianxiety meds for stress and lack of sleep—all have addictive potential. Even cough syrups and allergy medicines can cause certain withdrawal problems in many patients.

Unfortunately, what many doctors don't discuss with patients before prescribing these powerful drugs is the difficulty with withdrawal, even in drugs not considered potentially addictive. What I mean by this is that the real danger is how one stops taking these drugs. It is a subtle, subversive addiction, at first mental, and progressively incorporating physical dependence. And the dependence can happen more rapidly and subtly than any of us had ever suspected—sometimes literally after the first dose!

The latest data supports this: The percentage of outpatient medical visits that led to a prescription for the commonly used medications Valium, Ativan, and Xanax doubled from 2003 to 2015.

While the class of drugs this includes are mostly prescribed for anxiety, insomnia, and seizures, the study found that the biggest rise in prescriptions during this time period was for back pain and other types of chronic pain.

In fact recent studies have shown that just one course of opioids after surgery or an episode of acute pain can lead to a lifetime of addiction. There appears to be a linear curve that shows the addictive potential exists after a few days and increases with each week they are used. By four weeks of use, up to 40 percent of patients are addicted and can take a year or more to get off them. Further, early on, people develop a psychological craving to go back to these medications when pain of any kind returns.

Yes, sometimes these medications are necessary, but the less exposure a patient has, the less likely it is that the patient will become addicted.

And if this is not enough to make you think about alternatives for you and your loved ones, consider this. In the past five years, because of the mounting pressure on physicians to *not* prescribe pain medications, the number of prescriptions for opioids has decreased by 50 percent. Doctors are afraid to give patients these medications, even when needed, partly out of concern for their addictive potential, and partly because new laws are demanding that less of them be prescribed. So having an alternative seems to make sense!

Pain is, in many cases, short-lived or self-limiting, but other problems such as depression, anxiety, and psychological pain, as well as sleep disorders, often related to real-world stresses, are substantially harder to treat. This is because when people try to decrease their dose of their antidepressant and mind-numbing medications they feel worse, especially those who have become dependent on them, because when going off these drugs without another coping method, the sadness and pain increase, making withdrawal all the more difficult.

The medically and scientifically grounded truth is that we are not doomed to lives filled with pain, sadness, or suffering. Our bodies know how to heal themselves; our minds know how to decrease pain or discomfort and lessen the sense of crisis in our lives. It's simply a matter of remembering to take the time to take care of you. We need to slow down and recall how life was in childhood, before we were aware of life's stresses. It never occurs to a young child that she should interrupt her play and fun time because of a bruise or a bump; instead, it's a few tears and then back to the fun. Children are protected by the body's innate ability to take care of the pain through its own hormonal medication—and I can teach you to access that any time you want, and perhaps even to relax a little, not a bad alternative in my book!

So what is the solution? The addition of a simple, easy-to-learn technique I can teach you...through a simple, effective, and predictable method that is time-proven and guilt-free.

I am not saying that the solutions in this book are the easiest way out. It's obvious that popping a pill is quicker and gives a temporary sense of relief, or at least escape—but not the cure and not without consequences.

CHAPTER 2

'Ve combined preparation for surgery and the treatment of pain with the understanding that we are addressing the opioid crisis from inception to solution. As we have already seen, the path to opioids, addiction, and the difficulties of withdrawing from these medications is often directly tied to surgery or an injury that results in a prescription for as little as a single course of opioids.

This propensity to addiction is not a matter of toughness, lack of will, or lack of control of mind over body—it is a physiological process. The fact is, once the body gets a taste of the synthetic high, it craves it. The pleasure centers of the body, when stimulated, as per the work of Candace Pert, clearly show that the body craves feeling good. However it can get there, whatever it takes, the desire—and it's a strong one—is to go in that direction. Dr. Peart showed that the most common receptor on every cell in the body is the opioid receptor! That is correct; we are preprogrammed to desire and in fact strive for pleasure. This is a good thing if it is natural, but as with all good things, too much, especially if artificially created, is not necessarily better. For example, in the case of synthetic opioid abuse, it's harmful.

Patients who are in pain, who have suffered injuries, who have a need for relief from suffering whether it be mental or physical, will appropriately seek relief. This may come in many offered forms—injections, medications, and surgery, either one at a time or in combination. Couple this with the fear and anxiety associated with medical procedures and/or surgeries, along with the fear of sleeplessness and what is perceived as a worst-case scenario—the pain not going away—and we set up an anxiety, pain, and stress loop that is just looking for a cure. This loop in the brain feeds on itself—anxiety, spasms, heightened awareness of even minor discomforts, fear of worsening, and back to anxiety and stress over not gaining relief. If the first, and in many cases only, cure offered is drugs, the body and mind latch onto that with the addictive potential of a heroin addict.

So as a healer, a surgeon who treats patients with severe nerve pain and orthopedic pain, I have seen and agree with the literature. Treat the source from the beginning; avoid the apple from the garden of Eden: the drugs themselves—from the start, if at all possible. Sometimes it is as simple as the doctor or a nurse sitting down and explaining why a person is feeling symptoms and reassuring him or her that relief is coming, sooner than later. If people (that is correct, patients are people and the system often forgets that) have the tools we will talk about below to handle pain, anxiety, injury, or surgery, then less medication, easier healing, and happier lives prevail!

CHAPTER 3

Healing, Pain Control, and Surgery

Healing is all in your mind—and your mind is the most powerful healer you will ever encounter. I work with patients from every walk of life, including painters, artists, musicians, postal workers, nurses, doctors, window washers, bricklayers, billionaires, and paupers. Despite their outer differences, each of them has the same innate capacity to oversee and control the physiology of his or her own body. I've also learned that almost all medical challenges can be met by simply understanding that healing comes from within. And as a surgeon, I can tell you from someone who has seen it live, we are all the same inside. We all have the same beautiful colors, same-shaped organs, and same nervous systems, and we all heal the same way.

This is not just a book; it is a tool. The book comes with a healing, very powerful, extraordinarily effective audio portion that allows you to be in control of your pain, medical challenges, and even a situation where you thought you had none—the operating room. You control how your body reacts to, approaches, endures, and heals pain and injury, and even your body's reactions while asleep in surgery. I can teach you, as I have thousands of patients, to prepare yourself for dealing with pain, or the experience of surgery, change your actual physiology, and begin to heal even before your operation.

Medical research tells us—through PET, MRA, and MRI scans of the brain as well as testing of patients under anesthesia, in pain, and with sleep disorders as well as during operations—that the state of mind of the patient exerts extraordinary control over their physiological response to pain, surgery, and in fact every aspect of our lives. This is not a book about hope or wishing to get better; it is rather a guide that teaches you very simple techniques and behaviors that make discomfort and suffering fade and even disappear, sleep return to restful, and dealing with your important event and even surgery seem like simply a nap. So if you are having surgery, a dental procedure, facing stress or medication challenges, or even just looking to get a good night's sleep, this is a tool to get there in an enjoyable, comfortable, and yes, even fun way—to create your own personal healing agenda.

As Buddha said...it is all about control! In the case of healing or dealing with pain, once we give up that conscious control, our subconscious will gladly take over and make our desire to heal and be pain free a reality.

CHAPTER 4

How Will This Work

The audio portion that comes with this book is something very special. For those using these techniques to treat an already-present problem, such as dealing with pain or trying to wean from opioids, the techniques should be incorporated into your daily routines along with a coordinated program to find safe ways to decrease your medications with input from your doctor. For those facing an upcoming procedure, surgery, or life event that is challenging, the chapters are preparatory for getting ready for the day.

You will be given the opportunity to train your brain simply by listening to the first sessions a few times, either during your healing planning or before the day of your surgery. You will see how simple it is to prepare your body and mind to harness their phenomenal powers to heal and breeze through the day of your operation or handle your discomfort.

The follow-up audios allow you to either relax and listen on the day of surgery, or if your challenge is pain or sleep dysfunction, you'll begin to change that experience from the very beginning, attaining hope and early-yet-incremental improvements in dealing with these. The results can be dramatic. In the case of surgery, from the time you reach the hospital, you will begin feeling relaxed, happy, and blissful, and awaken after the operation relieved that you made all the difference in your own healing and experience. As you have listened and prepared yourself regularly beforehand, your subconscious mind will know and understand that this is the natural course that will ensue. With sleep or pain suffering, you will begin to feel control over your disease, addiction, or stressful daily challenges, and find the correct path to healing that is ideal for you as an individual.

CHAPTER 5

What Is Pain?

B uddha also said, "It's all about suffering."
We all gain the understanding of how to deal with suffering in one form or another. Without experiencing suffering, we would not grow stronger or be motivated to make changes in our lives, to strive for better, or know when something is wrong with our bodies.

In short and the truth—pain is your friend. It is your body's way of telling you that something is wrong or what you are doing is harmful.

Unfortunately our reaction to pain is what generally gets us in trouble, both as patients and physicians. When fear of pain becomes overwhelming, or people are not given appropriate coping mechanisms for their pain, the stress of preparation for surgery, injury, or psychological pain, bad things can happen. Dependency or rash decisions to have surgery are generally a result of no alternatives, or at least no perceived alternatives, and therefore a desperate attempt to get rid of pain, which leads to a vicious cycle. I am offering an alternative to exactly this situation, one that is easy and effective!

CHAPTER 6

What Exactly Is the Opioid Crisis and How Did We Get There?

Doctors by their very natures are nurturers. They strive to help people and to take their pain away. In fact the basis of the medical profession is to help relieve patients of their suffering and pain, ideally to heal whatever it is that ails them.

Unfortunately, long gone are the days when your family physician had time to make house calls, sit with you for forty-five minutes, and find out what really is making you suffer, including all the things that are going on in your life that might contribute to how you feel, your sadness, your stresses, and the resultant headache that won't go away because there is so much fighting and screaming in the household. I had a patient years ago who was not sleeping at night, and we tried everything to get her some relief. She related that she was just too uncomfortable and that her neck, back, and shoulder hurt. I sat and spoke with her one day and she related that her sleep issue might somehow be helped if only they "could get that car removed." I didn't quite understand, but as we chatted, she told me that they lived on a busy corner which cars came around very fast, and it seems one night instead of making the turn, a car drove straight up her front lawn and into the living room. From there ensued a significant dispute between the driver's auto insurance and the homeowner's insurance company. Neither would accept responsibility for the vehicle that sat in her living room along with the hole in the wall of her house. The car stayed there through this very cold winter, and she had no heat. The only place warm enough for her and her family to sleep was a cold floor in the farthest back room of the house. Once I understood and we got the car removed, we solved the sleep problem. We also solved much of her pain problem. Yes, it was a more lengthy, perhaps unforeseen answer to an orthopedic pain and sleep problem, but knowing her life circumstances was very helpful in getting her some relief and avoiding surgery.

Today, patients are not afforded the luxury of sharing their stories or their personal pains.

They are essentially the victims of a system that allows thirty seconds of conversation between patient and doctor. The doctor, well-meaning and wanting to help, gives the patient something that will give relief. These may be antidepressant medications or opioid painkillers to help the pain. Unfortunately in most cases it's simply a quick fix rather than actually understanding that problem and finding less dangerous solutions that are equally, if not more, effective, all because in many cases, the underlying cause of that suffering would be impossible to uncover in the limited time allotted for patient/doctor visits.

What seemed to be a good concept—efficiency through medication—unfortunately has led to today's opioid crisis. Little did anyone realize the severe addictive potential of these medications and the side effects on the body—not to mention the very real and destructive effects on society itself.

One of the first things we need to do is change our lifetime beliefs. You have been taught, programmed, and indoctrinated into the fallacy that the medical system and doctors take care of you. You do not take care of yourself if you get sick, you are anxious, you have a question, or you simply don't feel well; you need an "expert" to tell you how you feel and how to make it better. You've done your best to stay healthy, but without the doctor to tell you you're OK, you're not sure. You're told to get regular cancer screenings, checkups, and blood pressure checks, and take your medications as directed. It just isn't true.

Medicine is big business. In fact more than 30 percent of the working population of the United States is employed in one way or another in the medical field. It is almost impossible to break the dogma that we need doctors and medicine to be OK. And that's really fine. There are times when you need a doctor. Break a bone in two pieces and it's sitting sideways; you need a surgeon to put it back in the right position. Yes, your body will heal it, and yes, your bone will heal, but it would be nice to have it lined up. On the other hand, do you really need someone to tell you that you are OK? If you feel good, chances are you're probably OK.

We become addicted, not just to the medications we're given, not just to the reaching into the cabinet for medicine, a fix, or the like; we've become addicted to being taken care of. We've forgotten that we know how to take care of ourselves.

It all comes down to this: your mind is the most powerful healing tool that you have. It can make you feel great and make you feel lousy. All you need to do is program it and it can overcome any beliefs or long-term traditions. Intuitively you know what to do; these techniques are just giving you permission and a little bit of direction on how to be in charge of you.

We now live in a time when overdoses, drug interactions, depression secondary to medications, and suicides have resulted in a decreasing life expectancy, despite having the greatest medical technology available in the history of mankind. This inverse curve is in great part because we are not helping people heal their pain by giving them options other than medications to deal with their real-life pain and stress problems. Instead we are slowly poisoning our society in the name of efficiency due to a loss of humanity in the healing profession.

This is not just a problem for the patients; it is a problem for the healers as well. The statistics clearly show that doctors, nurses, and medical professionals are suffering severe burnout due to the stresses of having become technicians and pill pushers rather than healers who have relationships with their patients. There are no easy answers to this geopolitical dilemma...but there are answers for you! Hence the opioid alternative.

Georgia's Story

While treating her, I got to know Georgia well. Because of a terrible injury, she was devastated physically and emotionally and became a victim of her depression as well as the medications that had been prescribed for her. This was an extraordinarily positive and motivated lady who loved people and life, except for one issue: She had become addicted to Ativan, a mind-altering sleep medication that at first seemed harmless enough but soon became a literal nightmare.

I introduced Georgia to the techniques in this book and had a visit with her for followup the following December.

I recall chatting together about her very colorful Christmas outfit, right down to the flowered red shirt, green pants, and perfectly matched red glasses. She was the picture of the season, a happy person who was not only moving ahead with her life after the injury that had changed her world forever, but also was excited about this new chapter of her life.

What had changed from when I first met her and began caring for her was the question I could not help but ask. She shared with me that she had been using Ativan to sleep for many years and was frustrated at her inability to stop taking this medication; she was clearly addicted. She had tried to stop multiple times but basically found herself hopelessly dependent on the drug, incapable of falling asleep without it. As part of the treatment for her severe pain, we had Georgia learn medical meditation and relaxation techniques, and I also gave her a copy of my earlier book on meditation and self-hypnosis, *A Surgeon's Self-Hypnosis Healing Solution: My Father's Secret.*

My father's story of self-healing triggered something deep in her mind: the knowledge that she had the strength to relax herself, for sleep as well as to heal her pain. Georgia undertook learning medical meditation with full commitment and completely stopped the Ativan. She relates that she's sleeping wonderfully, and without the medications, her normal dream cycle has been restored, which has made her life even happier.

Indeed, the opioid alternative is not simply a different drug or trick; it is a path that helps you take back your life, making it happier and richer in every way.

CHAPTER 7

Who Has Surgery? Who Has Pain?

Almost everyone living today in the United States, in fact in the civilized world, will sometime or another face injury, a painful event, or a medical procedure of some kind: an operation, dental procedure, orthopedic procedure, diagnostic test, or major surgery. This certainty crosses all lines of race, money, occupation, and ages. The fact is, there are times when surgery is necessary and indeed it helps people to heal and get better. While I'm a strong advocate of first seeking conservative and alternative treatments, I know that surgery is, at times, absolutely the right decision—after all, I'm a surgeon and I know that, when necessary, it does help cure people. I believe that medication and opioids also have their place, although they can also lead to pain or sadness. So yes, I do recommend medication for some issues, and yes, I do operate on patients, and most of my patients do well when they have surgery. And those who are given medications benefit from them as well when they're used appropriately and ideally augmented with meditation and therapy techniques. My results are pretty good, in fact often great. It is not because I'm a superior surgeon; I just have superior patients! I say this in all honesty.

Our patients work with me in developing their treatment goals and plans, but most importantly are generally in agreement that it is good sense as well as good medicine to try everything reasonably possible before having an operation and or medication. If all else does not work and they understand the benefits and risks, then surgery or medication, used appropriately, are reasonable choices. The key to their successful outcomes is that they are prepared for the operation well before it takes place. And most importantly, they know how to relax. I feel so strongly about this that I request that every patient I operate on learn relaxation techniques and medical meditation, which is a form of self-hypnosis. They do better with the operations, feel better, heal better, require less pain medication and anesthesia, and if nothing else, they learn how to relax!

My Father's Secret: Medical Meditation

My father, a clinical psychologist who specialized in hypnosis, had five heart attacks - his first at forty-seven years of age, the last at fifty-two and cardiac bypass surgery which failed. His heart cardiac catheterization showed he had none of the original vessels remaining. He used medical meditation and self-hypnosis to "self-heal" and grow new vessels in his heart, which kept him alive. He lived a full life using the techniques he taught me and I offer here in these pages to you. He enjoyed over twenty years of happy and productive life using the power of his mind. Until about a year or two before he died, you would not have known on meeting him that he was debilitated. Never underestimate your ability to control your physiology—indeed you always do, you just don't know it!

What I want you to learn here is simply one thing—how relaxation and hypnotic self-suggestion specifically allow you to decrease pain and discomfort as well as have an operation successfully and comfortably and have a great result! I want you to understand what I have come to know as a surgeon, and I want you to know that as quickly and easily as possible.

What you will learn is simply the best, most effective, and extraordinarily easy way to prepare yourself for dealing with pain or injury, and when necessary, to undergo and successfully benefit from the surgery that you have chosen to have. I've used these methods for over a quarter of a century to help patients endure painful injuries, sleep disruption, come off or decrease medications, augment or avoid the need for opioid medications, and have successful, healing surgery.

Whether your primary motivation is to overcome your fear of going to the operating room, use less anesthesia, feel better when you wake up, or enhance your healing, you will achieve your goal. This method works. I will teach you a tool that you can use when you face any stressful or difficult situation—whether it's surgery, a broken arm, a dental procedure, or even headaches or stomach cramps. It is as predictable and reproducible as saying your name. The only difference is that saying your name doesn't always make you feel this good. I share with you now these easily learned and highly effective secrets. If you follow the directions I give you and stick with the plan, it's as simple as taking a nap!

CHAPTER 8

There Is Nothing New under the Sun—a Little History

This is really old news. Relaxation techniques and hypnosis are not new concepts for the management of pain and having surgery. In fact it wasn't that long ago that all we had to help patients in surgery was a shot of whiskey and a bullet to bite! That is also why the death rate for surgery in the 1800s was almost 80 percent.

Surgeons have known since the 1800s that surgical patients do better when they are relaxed and that in fact many do not even need deep anesthesia. In fact the use of hypnosis in Europe goes back many decades. James Esdaile, a Scottish surgeon who lived in the mid 1800s, had an astounding success rate with his surgeries; twice as many of his patients survived as compared to other surgeons. Esdaile learned to use hypnosis and relaxation techniques in India. He brought this knowledge back from Calcutta and in 1845 began using it for surgical anesthesia. By 1851 he had performed several thousand operations using hypnosis alone, and three hundred of these were major, life-threatening surgeries.

The advent of anesthesia brought with it some wonderful advances and indeed the use of anesthesia is something we are all entitled to. That said, anesthetics have complications and side effects, so using less and having fewer complications or side effects is a wonderful thing.

In 1843 John Elliotson published the results of seventy-six surgeries where hypnosis was the sole anesthetic. Surprisingly this was met with conflict among the medical society, even though most operations were performed in those days without anesthesia. It was not until 1846 that ether and then chloroform were discovered and used for anesthesia. After these drugs were adopted by the medical society, the teaching and use of hypnosis and relaxation techniques to anesthetize patients for surgery began to decline, even though the drugs had side effects and the hypnosis had none. Certainly medications were helpful and could have been used together with hypnosis, but the "quick fix of the ether" was too hard for the medical community and the public to resist, despite many complications from the anesthesia as well as actual chemical dangers in the operating room. The real sin was that the other benefits of hypnosis and relaxation, such as decreased anxiety, decreased need for medication, and improved post-op outcomes and attitudes were lost in the push for drugs—a harsh reminder of how opioid epidemics begin.

In 1848 Elliotson described perhaps the first-known application of hypnosis with cancer (not just for pain or surgery), pre-dating the more recent work in this area by approximately one hundred thirty years. The middle-aged woman was diagnosed by several prominent physicians as having breast cancer, which was felt by some of them to be inoperable. She was a deep-trance subject, and Elliotson used mesmerism, the original term for meditation and hypnosis, with her up to three times a day. She steadily progressed and gained weight and strength, her skin healed, and the tumor decreased in size. Curiously, when Elliotson traveled out of the country, the patient lost ground, but she continued to improve once he returned. He continued to use mesmerism with her for over five years with no sign of the return of the cancer in follow-up examinations by several physicians. When she died from a separate disease, inflammation of the lungs, the autopsy found no trace of cancer!

Dr. Corydon Hammond, a clinical psychologist and specialist in neurofeedback, in his paper "Review of the Efficacy of Clinical Hypnosis with Headaches and Migraines," defines options to medication provided through the healing aspects of the patient/physician partnership as well as hypnosis.

Dr. Bernie Siegel, in his book *Love, Medicine and Miracles*, shares many stories of patients healing from their cancer diagnoses through belief in the outcomes of chemotherapy and surgery. He teaches that the mind is very powerful, and how we see these as healing interventions as opposed to "chemicals that kill or knives that cut" makes all the difference in how the body reacts to them. Healing is very much in the mind, and he has hundreds of stories that bear this out.

Although relaxation, medical meditation, and hypnotic self-suggestion have also been used in modern times as the sole anesthesia, in major operations I often suggest a combination approach as the best option for many. In my experience it is often best used to augment the use of less medication, together with modern techniques such as sedation anesthesia or local anesthesia. This means you get all the benefits of the chemical anesthesia while using a much smaller dosage, with minimal if any side effects, equal or better control of discomfort and relaxation, and feeling great afterward.

With my patients who have surgery, I use the fact that people hear under anesthesia to their benefit. I have them listen to an audio during the surgery of these same medical meditations, giving positive thoughts and healing suggestions—while your conscious mind is asleep, your subconscious is awake, taking care of you! This results in less stress, lessening of side effects or discomfort postoperatively, less need for medications after surgery, and faster healing—all by simply relaxing a little!

Surgeons

Surgeons are an interesting group. We are trained to do things to you to heal you—and some of these can be unpleasant! It's not that surgeons are bad or sadistic people; in fact, surgeons are generally a pretty helpful group. If you need something done, and it needs to get done in a technically excellent way, many surgeons can do that. But by the very nature of their profession, surgeons have ingrained in them the ability to manifest emotional detachment. By this I mean that although they care about you, they really can't get emotionally involved when they are visualizing and thinking about what they do. Essentially they are cutting your body open and must have a certain frame of mind and reference to do that. Most surgeons are not "touchy-feely" people, and they spend a lot of time learning about the technical aspects of surgery. This means that often during training, there is not a great deal of time spent on how the patient feels (or frankly, how we feel) when going through the experience.

This was highlighted by a very funny conversation (at least one of us found it amusing) I had with our youngest daughter when she was in high school. She had asked about medical school and was briefly considering the possibility of becoming a surgeon. She is a very detail-oriented person, now an electrical and computer as well as software engineer, who's very skilled in visualizing and creating—important for a surgeon. But I unwittingly focused on what in my mind was a great asset she also exhibited: the capacity for detached compassion! This is an essential component for a surgeon, allowing her to violate another person's body but see it as an act of healing. Well, this was not taken lightly by my daughter, who saw it more as an insult than compliment. It made me rethink whether we surgeons (myself included) should have more insight into feelings and not simply become mechanics.

CHAPTER 9

The Secret Surgeons and Healers Don't Tell You

I've presented and taught these relaxation techniques to surgeons and doctors at meetings of the American Society of Clinical Hypnosis, the equally prestigious American Association for Hand Surgery, and the Academy for Orthopaedic Surgeons.

What I will share with you here is the inside scoop. We surgeons know that the challenge of surgery is not having or surviving it. Thousands of people have surgery every day and in fact essentially every one of us will have one or more operations during our lifetime. And most people do just fine. The tragedies are sensationalized and many times when things go awry, it is related to stress imposed (unintentionally, but as a byproduct of the process) on the patient, both physiologic and psychological. But most often, surgery is not that difficult of a process. What is difficult, mentally challenging and highly stressful is this: the stress of deciding if you should have surgery, getting there, and going through the procedure. Once we overcome our anxiety and decide to proceed (meaning before deciding to go to surgery, we have soul-searched the decision and options), most operations go just fine!

Years ago I had a patient, Ralph, and he was quite a guy. He was an entrepreneur and a very successful businessman. He told me something that I have never forgotten. He had a significant problem with one of the nerves in his arm and needed surgery. I had tried most everything with him to avoid surgery, but medically the logical decision was that he needed to have an operation. He had seen other doctors but chose me to do his surgery.

When we talked about what I considered a very difficult decision for him as we sat face to face in my exam room, I looked him in the eyes and said, "Ralph, yours is a very tough seat to be in. It's difficult to make these decisions."

He locked his eyes on mine and said, "No, yours is the harder seat."

I questioned him, "Why?"

Ralph said, "Listen, I'm a guy who makes lots of decisions every day. I judge things, make tough choices, and judge the benefits and risks. I've researched you, and I know about you. I know your reputation, your statistics, and that you're a good surgeon and a nice guy. I know that you've done this operation and know much more about the right choice than I do. Therefore I made my decision."

He then explained: "I do all the research I can concerning any decision I make that is important. I check out the experts but evaluate them as people and the nature as best I can of the problem, then I talk to them. Once I've determined fully the challenge and the choices, I try the most conservative and simple options first. If further action is required, I know I have found someone I trust and who knows as much as can be known about the problem—then I turn over the control to them. I can then relax and let things happen."

This is what Ralph did with me. He had the operation and did wonderfully. Not a peep, not a problem, and he went on to have a normal life.

What Ralph taught me is that being in control is a wonderful thing, and when you have control of your mind and body and your decision process, there are times when the right decision is to give up control. Once you know whom to give up the control to, then you are in good shape. You maintain control of the decision process right up to the point where you turn it over to a person better qualified. This is no different than being in an airplane. Unless you are a certified, licensed pilot, you're likely going to turn over control to the pilot even before you step on board, rather than trying to fly yourself. You've already turned over control to the airline because you know they will make a better choice and supply excellently trained pilots for you. It is a conscious decision and a good one based on all of what we discussed above.

The above insights hold equally true for surgery or when dealing with pain and injury. Stress increases pain; it heightens the intensity of nerve impulses and perception of pain. It also causes muscle spasms and because muscles surround nerves, increased muscle spasms squeeze the nerves and increase their pain intensity even further. Stress also increases your sympathetic response, the stress response thereby heightening the intensity of the pain even more.

Anxiety and stress are the most substantial generators of pain and suffering in most people; in fact, 90 percent of office visits are shown to be for stress-related or stress-induced complaints. Pain is real, but suffering is a choice, at least to some extent its intensity. The degree of suffering can be lessened by learning simple techniques that allow you to relax and use your body's own chemicals to decrease pain, be it emotional or physical. This is a hard pill to swallow, if you will allow the purposeful play on words, but a truism. All of us know that even when we are in pain or suffering in some way, the degree and level of this changes regularly, from different times of day, cold or hot weather, what we are doing, or what we are thinking. So the solution becomes a relatively straightforward one—find the triggers to what is increasing it, find the releases that exist, even if temporary, and begin training your mind to change its focus, and yes, its perception of that pain. This is achievable in almost all cases and predictable.

Remember also that your doctor feels the same stresses, and many silently suffer with you. Doctors constantly must make decisions, prescribe medications and procedures, and read your test results and interpret them. Then they must decide what treatment and direction for your care will be the best for you. This hopefully means they take *you* into the equation—your unique strengths, fears, other medical issues, and your preferences as to what you are comfortable with.

For your doc, nurse, therapist, or other medical professional, each decision can possibly have real, long-term, and even life-changing consequences—so the pressure to get it right or at least make the best choice every time is tremendous. Doctor burnout is a real thing, a result of the stresses of each decision they make all day long.

So here is the secret:

Surgeons and docs fear one thing more than anything else:

A bad result!

It is not a personal thing; surgeons have egos, like all of us, but with a catch. You see, it takes a very different mindset and personality to allow them to boldly cut open a fellow human and believe they are going to heal them! The same holds true for doctors making a diagnosis and implementing a treatment plan or giving medications to save a life or decrease pain and suffering.

Yes, it takes a pretty big ego, but in most cases, it is not a God complex, but I will tell you it takes a specific amount of chutzpah to do it. And a doctor/surgeon is only as good as her last operation or last good call. In other words we are people too, and we know we are not perfect. We are influenced by our moods, the people we are working with, the way we feel that day, and yes, the faith of our patients.

So here is the rub, a way to hedge your bets for a happy and healthy process: When you are calm and approach your surgery and doctor in the way I will teach you, it will make your doctor a better surgeon, you a better patient, and your operation or choice of treatments a success!

CHAPTER 10

Why Do You Make Them Wait, Paul? Why?

I trained with a wonderful surgeon many years ago at the University of Pennsylvania. I was a young resident, learning to do joint replacement surgery. His specialty was knee operations and replacements. Paul was one of the best. His technical skills were only outdone by his people skills. I would sit in the exam room with him as he evaluated and spoke with patient after patient. They came with canes, walkers, and wheelchairs. Many were so debilitated it was beyond my understanding why they had not been operated on long before. The art of joint replacement surgery was relatively young, and the implants were still in development phase. Some worked very well, but there were definitely (as there are still) complications with some of these surgeries. Many patients did well with the operations, but others developed problems such as loosening and breakage of the implants, infections, and even loss of legs. These complications are still possible today, but in the early days they were even more so.

One day I asked Paul why he didn't operate on more of these people. Why did he make them wait? He told me something I've never forgotten. He said: "Scott, these people need to understand the serious nature of the operation. They need to reach a point where they really understand what they want and why they want it. The operation will not cure them all; some will need other operations, and a reasonable number of them will do poorly. This operation will be a partnership, and our patients need to be part of the decision and make an informed choice about their bodies. They need to remember the suffering they had to endure so they will truly appreciate the improvement. We cannot make them normal; we can only hope to improve their lives. They also need to know that if they do not get better, they tried everything else first."

Years later I came to understand that there were two lessons here:

One: that the people having operations or dealing with injuries, pain, or life crises could help make a difference in the operation's outcome.

Two: when we visualize something, when we see the result and when we *really* want it, a more successful outcome is likely. This is visualization, imagery, and hypnosis. This was why his patients did better. I've tried to live my professional life by these words. I always want my patients to partner with me in making decisions about operations, therapies, medications, and treatment alternatives. If they decide to use medications or invasive treatments or to have an operation, this choice is based on their understanding of their situation and that they've done everything to try to heal before opting for surgery, as well as knowing that no operation or surgeon is perfect. They clearly see and understand their choices and consciously choose the path. They must know in their own mind that this is what they really want and need to do.

Meditation and medical hypnosis allow people to know their own minds and use them to their advantage. In this book I can give you the tools to use your own mind—not only to make the right decision for you and your body but to be able to use less medication. Further, if it's surgery or an injury that requires extensive healing, I can help you improve the chances that your recovery will be the success you visualize.

CHAPTER 11

Wide-Awake Surgery... Excuse Me?

A 2011 article published in the *Journal of the American Association for Hand Surgery* titled "Wide-Awake Trapeziectomy" points out this lack of compassion among surgeons loud and clear. It prompted a trend and follow-up articles and techniques as well as seminars on performing "wide-awake surgeries." This is a technique touted as the upcoming rage in many countries and has been embraced recently here in the United States. Essentially what it means is exactly what it says. You're wide awake, they inject you and numb your hand up and operate on you.

They do not give any sedation or anesthesia except for numbing up the hand or area of operation. I believe personally that this is rather barbaric, and that no preparation or sedation of any sort is not fair to people. This is why many children who had procedures in the emergency room years ago have traumatic memories of doctors and medicine. They used to be strapped into something called a papoose and had procedures done with the thought that kids didn't have to be sedated and would "forget it" later in life. Trust me, these are things you and your children do not forget.

It seems to me a technique more from the 1800s than today. Can you imagine asking and promoting that a patient will have no anesthesia whatsoever, no ability to relax or escape from the anxiety and stress of the environment, and then have an operation? It's certainly not the way I want to be treated. It is, unfortunately, a telling sign of the coming future in "cost effective medicine." Fewer dollars are being spent to take care of people, and it seems the goal is to cost cut at the expense of the patient's comfort, eliminating the relaxation portion of the anesthesia. It is anesthesia with the goal of saving millions of dollars but unfortunately at the expense of patient comfort and at times the long term outcome of the surgical procedure. The bad news is that this is something that foretells the future of medicine and surgery in this country with the coming health care reforms; you can expect, at the very least, less general anesthesia and more sedation operations, and the worst, more fully wide-awake surgery.

I say all this not to scare you, and yes, you should speak with your surgeon and anesthesiologist to be sure the right combination of options is made available to you. What is a person to do? Everyone is different; some require more help with pain control than others, but certainly asking and discussing this preoperatively is appropriate and necessary. That said, if you are pressed and given little choice in the matter, at least if you learn these relaxation and mind-control techniques, you have an option that will help you be in control and either substitute for or enhance whatever limited options they offer. For those who embrace these techniques fully, it might even be an advantage since you awaken and feel great, not drugged. Again, my medical choice is to use both, medication in a dose that is correct for the patient but also medical meditation to enhance the effect and limit side effects. Cost should not be a factor when it comes to your personal health, and the added costs of a minimal amount of sedation are far outweighed by feeling better post operatively. Humanity must survive in medical care and, in a worst case scenario, at least you have the ability to help yourself! And here is another plus for learning what I am teaching you in this book; if for some reason medically you cannot have the medications, you have an alternative, and it is all in your control.

I offer here answers on how to easily do this—more on that later; you not only get to take care of you, but you will learn how to make the system work for you!

CHAPTER 12

What Is Medical Meditation?

So what is medical meditation or medical self-hypnosis, relaxation, and mindfulness? In essence this is a conscious commitment to live life fully, happily, and healthfully and to have control over your body, eliminate or lessen discomfort, and minimize the need for external stimulants, painkillers, or more aggressive and invasive medical treatments. This goes well beyond the concept of simply wanting to be healthy or feel good; it is a conscious process that creates health and well-being. Medical meditation puts your body in a state where every day, subconsciously, all day long, it goes about healing, regenerating, recuperating, and decreasing the intensity of the temporary fluctuations that cause us discomfort, either mental or physical. It is also about having enough respect and love for yourself to create a life that, through simple changes in behavior, allows you to eat more healthfully, be more relaxed, happy, and in the moment, and exercise just the right amount. Essentially, medical meditation gives you the power and control to care for you, your body, and your world in a very comfortable, relaxed, and enjoyable way.

Medical meditation is a technique that is complication-free and predictable! It is an alternative way of healing most disease processes, decreasing pain, limiting the need for medications, and dealing with life's traumas. With it you can reduce pain, improve sleep, decrease anxiety, and yes, when necessary, dream your way through medical procedures and surgery.

When we talk about meditation, relaxation, and hypnosis, we really are talking about self-hypnosis. Many people are under the misconception that someone else or even I can hypnotize you. In fact and reality, no one can hypnotize anyone. Hypnosis, meditation, mindfulness, and relaxation are all self-hypnosis. Only you can hypnotize yourself. Only you can relax yourself and this is what this is all about. These are not new techniques. The concepts of meditation, relaxation, and hypnosis go back to the ancient Egyptians, where they had actual healing rooms in their temples. The Assyrians, Aristotle, Hippocrates—all the great healers—knew the power of the human mind to heal itself. All you need do is understand how to bring yourself to that relaxed state, and you can manifest your own healing as well.

This relaxed state is not something that is new to you. You've known how to do it all your life. Basically it's called an alpha state. That is the state where your brain waves slow down just a bit. You've achieved this many times. Every night just before you drift off to sleep. If you remember way back when you got a good night sleep, you're lying there, drifting, thinking about the day, perhaps your next day, and all of a sudden you wake up and its morning. That state just before you fall asleep is the alpha state. That is the state you achieve when you do self-hypnosis or relaxation. All it really is, is a fixed focused state of concentration. You've done it many times, from daydreaming to intensely doing something you love.

So what is medical meditation or medical self-hypnosis? Simply stated, **it is the absolute positive belief that a fixed focused state of concentration will allow the body's innate capacity for healing to manifest.** What I mean by this is that if you focus specifically on healing, on feeling good, it has no choice but to manifest.

Have you ever been in a room, and someone yawned? Pretty soon you get the urge, and you yawn. This is a hypnotic suggestion. Or someone sitting next to you's stomach begins to grumble. Pretty soon your stomach begins grumbling, and you become hungry and want to eat as well. This is your subconscious mind picking up a nonverbal influence, a primal suggestion. These are forms of self-hypnotic suggestion. The same concept allows you to drive somewhere and not even remember the trip! You might get there and don't even remember what you thought about or wonder where the time went. You call it daydreaming, but you were still focusing and driving. That's a hypnotic state, a fixed, focused state of concentration.

Or what about going to a movie? While you're in the theater, you're living that movie; you're crying with these people or perhaps rooting for your hero. You're completely involved in that scene, in that movie, in that reality. It is an altered state of reality that you've placed yourself in. The movie doesn't put you there; you place yourself in it, fully and completely being part of it all. That again is a self-hypnotic state. And when you leave the theatre, you blink your eyes. You're not really adjusting to the light. You're readjusting your mind, coming back, literally, to reality and out of your altered state.

Children are natural meditators and daydreamers; they have no problem blending fantasy and reality. As a surgeon I have treated many children who've accidentally had car doors closed on their little fingers. Often when they get to the ER, the finger is bleeding. It is swollen, and in some cases, even partially amputated. Understandably, many times the child (and often the parent) is crying uncontrollably—hysterically. Usually if at all possible I'll say, "Hey, look at that."

They're like, "What?"

I repeat to them, "Look at that, over there."

Again through the sobs I eventually hear them say, "Look at what? I don't see anything."

And I say, "That, right there. Look at that." It may be a funny shirt that nurse is wearing or some other object that is a little unusual; it really does not matter. As long as the child is focused over there, on anything other than the finger, at that moment, in their mind, this injured finger doesn't exist. I can fix the finger, suture it back on, put a pin in it to stabilize the bone if I need to, and as long as that child is looking over that fixed point, this finger doesn't exist. Full disclosure: I generally use this technique for getting them calm and performing examinations, and once we can work with them we add little additional anesthetic to perform any real surgical procedures. But it helps to have the child and parents calmer to make good decisions and have better outcomes. This is the beauty of the state of focused concentration - when that one thought in your mind is focused in one area; this finger, or whatever else is a problem, doesn't exist.

The Conscious and Subconscious Minds

You see your mind is very busy. It's divided into two parts: the conscious and subconscious. Your conscious mind is the mind that is aware of everything that's going on. It's very, very busy, in fact it processes seventeen trillion pieces of information a second. How's the light in this room? That picture on the wall—it's a little crooked. Maybe that color on that carpet could be a little different. Where is my arm sitting? What does this chair feel like on my back? Am I postured correctly? It is very, very, very busy. It takes care of our day-to-day business of living. Unfortunately it also makes us a little crazy sometimes. This is our conscious mind.

The other part of our mind is the subconscious, the part of our mind that takes care of us. The beauty of the subconscious mind is that without even being aware of it, this baby makes sure your basic physiology stays healthy. For instance, when is the last time you sat and said, "Heart—beat one, beat two, beat three"? Of course you don't have to do that. Your subconscious mind knows to make your heart beat sixty beats a minute, sixty minutes an hour, twenty-four hours a day for your whole life. And, in times of increased need, such as exercise or physical exertion, it makes your heart beat faster and with stronger ejection strength of the blood, as needed for that situation without you having to give that a thought.

The same holds true for your breathing. You don't say, "Breath in…breath out." No, you don't have to do that. Only occasionally are you aware of your breathing, when something causes you to notice it. Your subconscious mind takes care of that. It knows how to take care of you.

Your subconscious mind also secretes hormones, very powerful hormones that control your body's function. Some of them are your feel-good hormones, the endorphins, the enkephalins, and serotonin. These hormones are the ones that take care of you, make you relaxed, and make you happy and feel good. Melatonin is another hormone secreted from your subconscious mind, which makes you sleep. So the great news is that when the subconscious mind is relaxed, and our conscious stresses stay out of its way, we are allowing it to take care of us, and it does exactly that!

The subconscious mind also knows how to heal your body. Let's say you have a cut on the back of your hand. You don't sit there and look at the cut and say, "All right, white cells, I want you to come in and make sure no infection occurs - and granulation tissue please begin the healing from the bottom up". You don't need to do any of that. You just need to let your subconscious mind secrete the right hormones, send the right messages to the area in need, and your body and its marvelous healing systems simply does its thing and heals you. The key is that your body heals better and feels better when you are in a relaxed state. Because when you are relaxed, your body is better able to do what it knows how to do without having to focus on calming down your stress.

Stressed out?

Let's talk for a few moments about stress. Stress begins, grows, and resolves in our minds. It is not a physical entity until we make it so by allowing it to affect our physiology simply by its existing.

Sure, we need some stresses to push us to jump out of the way of an oncoming car or maybe to motivate us to study for a test, and the stress of a lecture from our boss makes us do our job.

When you stop to think about it, this society rewards us for being stressed and stressed out. When is the last time your boss or your teacher told you, "I want you to do absolutely nothing today, nothing. I just want you to sit around do nothing. In fact I don't even care if you show up, and I'm going to double what I pay you." It doesn't happen. No one rewards you for relaxing, but this society rewards you for being stressed, and the more stressed you are, the more stressed out you get, the more rewarded you are. Ever walk through a parking lot and look at the handicapped spaces? They've often got the nicest cars in them, haven't they? Because these people worked themselves sick, something I refer to as the "work effect." They rewarded themselves, but they got there by ultimately ruining their own health.

CHAPTER 13

The Magic Painkiller

Way back behind your eyes, between your ears, and at the base of your brain is a small gland called the pituitary. You may want to imagine it as a small sponge. The pituitary gland contains all the chemicals and hormones that make your body heal and feel well. Yes, there are some other hormone-producing areas in the body, but let's focus on the pituitary. It produces chemicals such as endorphins, enkephalins, and serotonin. I call these the feel-good hormones. It also produces its own endogenous morphine. Morphine is the most powerful "happifier" or discomfort-reliever known to mankind. Simply squeezing a small drop of these hormones out into the bloodstream allows them to go to exactly the right place at exactly the right time. If you wish to feel happy and healthy with no discomfort at all through an operation, and awaken feeling happy, wonderful and relaxed, all you need to do is squeeze these hormones out into your bloodstream, and that is exactly what you will produce. The same holds true for a broken bone, dental procedure, or headache. It even gets better. You see, you don't have to think about squeezing any amounts out, figuring doses or exactly which hormones you need—your subconscious mind controls the pituitary. When you place an image in your mind of you being happy, healthy, and relaxed, having had a wonderful day and wonderful operation, you will achieve exactly that. No need for the conscious you to get involved in any way, except wishing to see yourself as happy, healthy, and relaxed. Once you begin to envision exactly what you want and how you want to feel, your body knows how to make that happen. Your subconscious mind responds to images. As long as you place the image of your health and happiness and your success with the surgery, that is all you need. It seems difficult to believe, but I've seen it time and time again with hundreds and hundreds of patients. The single factor you need is belief. Once you believe, truly believe, and understand that this is in your control and you can make it happen, it will!

CHAPTER 14

Let Me Teach You to Be a Parasympathetic Person

Your subconscious mind is divided into two portions: the sympathetic and parasympathetic nervous systems.

Have you ever heard of the fight-and-flight mechanism? It goes something like this: You are walking down an alley at one in the morning—it's very dark and eerily quiet—and suddenly someone jumps out from behind you and yells. You appropriately react, and your fight-or-flight mechanism begins to take over. Your heart rate increases, breathing gets faster, your pupils dilate, and your pores all open, with the hair standing up on your arms; this protective mechanism prepares you and your body to either fight or run (flight). This is a natural and essential protective mechanism for your body. This is your sympathetic nervous system at work; it is there to help you survive stressful or life-threatening situations, and it's very good at what it does when it is needed. The problem with this sympathetic mechanism is that in our days of too much stress, it often goes a little haywire, reacting to imagined/perceived threats rather than real ones. These come from everything—the daily news, overbearing bosses, relationships, and unfortunately for us all, our own imaginations.

Luckily your body has an equally effective and artfully skilled opposing mechanism called the parasympathetic nervous system. This too is the part of your neural/hormonal system, and its job is to balance the sympathetic nervous system. Its actions slow your heart rate and your breathing and decrease muscle spasms. It relaxes everything and lets it go.

Now although you are born with an equal ability to activate either system, unfortunately most of us have learned or been programmed through our society to be much more sympathetically active than parasympathetically so. Yes, you can consciously activate either the parasympathetic or sympathetic nervous system once you learn how, but for most of us, the sympathetic seems to be more easily stimulated; hence we are generally living in a higher-stress mode. This means we are more prone to stress and anticipation as well as reaction to pain.

The good news is that simply by slowing your breathing to less than eight breaths a minute you bring yourself to the alpha state, which increases the parasympathetic response and relaxes you. This is a natural protective mechanism of your body. Once you realize this and get in touch with your softer side, your calmer side, you begin to realize how to react in states of anxiety or stress. The body knows what to do, and if you just slow down, and slow down your breathing, it will occur quite naturally.

All that it takes to balance this is practicing relaxing. So if you practice getting calm and being relaxed, you get the expected physiologic response...your blood pressure lowers, your immune system calms down, and your blood pressure decreases, as do your cholesterol levels – as a result, there is less inflammation and irritation throughout your body and in your mind. By simply relaxing, your vessels open up and flow better, and the vessels heal as well as maintain their life-saving elasticity. Plaque, cholesterol buildup, and atherosclerosis actually reverse. What happens is, when the body learns to relax even for twenty minutes a day, it begins continuing this healing process, and this is the key to why medical meditation and relaxation techniques work. The parasympathetic nervous system remembers how to take care of your, the sympathetic response lessens, and the body heals.

CHAPTER 15

Let's Talk a Little about What Self-Hypnosis—or Medical Meditation—Is Not

This is not stage hypnosis. No one is going to get up on this desk and dance the hula or cluck like a chicken. You will never do anything in a state of hypnosis that you would not normally do in your regular waking state. You will never violate your morals, your ethics, or your religious beliefs. This is not a religious experience or anything like that. It is simply a state of relaxation.

The hypnotic state is something that will never harm you. It is risk free, complication free, and it cannot harm your body. Your subconscious mind has certain baseline protective mechanisms that will always take care of you. You can slow your heart rate, but you cannot stop your heart, because your subconscious knows that your heart must beat. You can slow down your breathing, and in fact it is good to slow your breathing, but you cannot stop yourself from taking a breath. You can never go into a hypnotic state, a sleep state, and not wake up. You will never bring yourself in and not be able to come out.

You cannot leave your body. Your soul is not involved in this. Your consciousness will always stay with you, so you can never leave your own sense of self or your own body.

The hypnotic state is just a relaxed state. It is a way to allow your body to work calmly and effectively.

The beauty of the subconscious mind is that it knows no difference between reality and fantasy. As long as it is something that will not harm you, and it is within the realm of reality, the subconscious mind will help you achieve it.

Let's say for instance you decide you'd like to have $10,000 in the bank. You say, "I think I'd like an extra $10,000." That wouldn't be bad, right? So every day you put yourself in your relaxed state, and you see that $10,000. You see yourself writing a check for that $10,000. You see yourself going on a shopping spree and enjoying that $10,000. That $10,000 is as real to your subconscious mind as my hand is right here in front of me. You'll meditate on this daily, and one day you'll wake up and say, "I've got it. I know how to do this. Every day on my way to work, I stop at one of those gourmet coffee places, and I buy myself a nice five-dollar cup of coffee, and in fact I've been liking them so much, I stop now twice a day." So every day you've been spending that money, and your subconscious says to you, "I think I'll stop." So you go and buy yourself a little coffee maker and make yourself a ten-cent cup of coffee every day. At the end of the week, you've saved yourself thirty-five dollars. At the end of the month, a hundred and twenty dollars. At the end of a year, $1,500, and pretty soon you have $10,000 in the bank, all by doing less. By relaxing. By not stressing out. By having less caffeine in your system. By doing nothing or less, you've made $10,000. And this is how the subconscious mind works; it filters. It gets an idea, and then it creates reality. And the subconscious mind works in images. It works in what we call the world of imagery. It sees things, and what it sees as reality, it creates.

So if your subconscious mind sees you as a happy, healthy, relaxed individual, that is what you become. Does it happen immediately? No. The subconscious mind works by secreting hormones and allowing you to change behavior patterns. If you are a person who, every time someone cuts off your car, yells and screams and jumps and loses it, eventually you'll be able to calm that down. Because you'll realize that it is harmful to you, and when you feel your blood vessels constricting and your stomach tightening and you become aware just by relaxing of what it's doing to you, you don't want to do that anymore. Or perhaps fried, fatty foods bother your stomach and digestion. Well, if you are aware and your subconscious is aware, you look at those foods and say, "I don't think I want to eat them." And you'll feel better. So this is how it begins to work when in your healing. As the subconscious mind has this image, it changes your physiology, enhances your healing, lowers your blood pressure, decreases muscle spasms, and increases the circulation and blood flow to your nerves, your tendons, your ligaments, and your muscles. It allows better healing. If you decide you want to be more physically fit, and you see yourself physically fit in your subconscious mind, you may eat slightly less. And you begin to achieve these realities because your subconscious mind sees them, and it really is that simple. It is so simple that we often miss the simplicity of it.

We've forgotten as a society that we are the ones who control our own minds. Whatever we decide our minds will think is what they will accept. It is your decision; it is your control. And by using simple techniques like this you gain the control, you gain the benefits, and you gain whatever reality you choose. Because in reality we control our minds, and our minds control our bodies.

Now, this is not a selfish pursuit. This is selfless. When you take care of you, you are less of a burden to those around you. When you have the ability to take care of you, your mind, and your body, you are better able to perform and achieve whatever you like. And when you better take care of yourself, you can take care better of those you care about. That is something that is very important to many people. Not only are you not a burden. Not only do you live life better. But you are better able to care for those you care about. What better gift in this world than taking care of you, taking care of those around you, and living life to its fullest?

When you consider the fact that our bodies regenerate themselves every seven years, that is, every seven years all of the cells in your body are replaced by new cells, you realize that you have the potential to recreate, repair, heal, and even make better any organ, muscle, nerve, or any portion of your body which you are unhappy with or which is not functioning the way you would like. So the benefit here is that if you are in a relaxed, happy, and healthy state and state of mind, the new cells that are going to be created are going to be happy cells, healthier cells. They are going to function better and feel better. Yes, as time goes on, you're going to have some bumps and bruises and dings, but the internal workings of your body can become even younger and better and healthier.

Over the past thirty years in my medical practice, I've had a chance to study people and see patterns in those who age best. They are the ones who have a healthy and happy outlook about life. They eat fairly well, do some exercise, and they meditate or relax—some are simply naturally happy people. These people live well into their seventies, eighties, nineties, and beyond, enjoying life, enjoying the day-to-day living because they feel good, and they have the right attitude. Further, when injuries occur or things set them back, they heal because they are mentally prepared to heal right. So this regeneration process, this repair process, is what our subconscious mind controls. And as long as the image is there in the subconscious mind that they are happy, healthy, relaxed, and feeling great, that's exactly what happens. And the process continues even when you are not thinking about it. You don't need to sit and meditate twenty-four hours a day to make the healing occur. You put the suggestion in your subconscious mind and just like that $10,000, it will manifest. It will appear. It will happen because your subconscious only knows how to please you. How to do what you see and what you want.

As a surgeon I can tell you with absolute positivity that these things are true. I have seen patients in the operating room who had hypertensive crises—where their blood pressure went up so high that we discussed cancelling the operation—consciously lower their blood pressure simply by using these techniques. I've seen them stop bleeding inside their bodies and make muscles soften and vessels begin to flow after they are repaired. Our patients go in and out of surgery with minimal if any discomfort, limiting their need for excessive amounts of anesthesia as well as requiring very little medication after surgery, even though they know they have it if they want it. All because they knew how to relax and help heal themselves. It's not that any of these individuals had any unusual skills or talents, each is no different than you or me. All they had was a tool to bring themselves to this relaxed state. Whether it's a swollen broken toe, lowering your cholesterol, or opening your cardiac blood vessels—whatever you choose to use it for, you can.

What we know universally is this: The human mind has tremendous capabilities. The smartest man who ever lived used twelve percent of his brain. The rest of our brains are the part that are incorporated through the subconscious, through the imagery. This portion of our brain does not need to be governed by us. It does not need to be used by us. All we need do to make this portion of our brain work is relax and take care of ourselves.

And the wonderful thing about medical meditation is that there are only three basic things that have to happen in order for this to work for you.

There are only three things that need to be in your mind in order for you to learn and use medical meditation and self-hypnosis:

1. *The first is that you have to want it. Well, you're here. You're reading this now. You have a need, a desire, the motivation.*

2. *The second is that you must practice it daily. Now some days you may not have twenty minutes, you may only have ten, and that's OK. But your body needs to get used to imparting the parasympathetic response. It needs to get used to relaxing again and know that this is natural.*

3. *And the third is that you must believe that this will work. You must believe that medical meditation and*

self-hypnosis is a powerful tool which will allow you to heal and be healthy.

Listen to Audio #1:
Here is your first Audio to introduce you to
medical meditation:

An Introduction to Medical Meditation
How to do your Medical Meditation

CHAPTER 16

Questions and Concerns Patients Share

Let's talk about a few of the challenges you will have from your own mind:

1. Fear of pain, surgery, and sickness!

Of course, the real fear about surgery isn't the operation itself; it is deeper, more primal. We are all afraid we're going to die during the operation, or it is going to hurt. Every single one of us. The same holds true for sickness or pain; I am certain most of us have heard someone say, "It hurts so much I feel like I am going to die." It is indeed the most primal fear we have, and an important one for our survival and to protect us—motivating action to alleviate the cause of the pain, or in some cases, such as an oncoming car while crossing a street, actual life-threatening danger. But when left to the imagination of "what might be," it can play on our emotions and create fear, anxiety, and actual physiological changes that become harmful rather than protective.

In fact the main thing that separates humans from all other species is our imagination. It is what allows us to put people on the moon, create art and literature, and thrive. But it can also become our own worst enemy when it runs wild and shows us the worst outcomes of daily situations, when in reality they are simply daily events, seen in a different light due to stories we may have heard, opinions we may have read, or prior similar experiences that did not go as well as hoped, either to us or someone we knew or loved. So when our fear and imagination become confused in the mind with logical thought, the challenge can become overwhelming. Hence, facing surgery, pain, cancer, or sleep-deprivation, we are often challenged by our own minds.

None of us is immune to this. I recall my own challenge years ago when our son Josh was very young. He had a common inguinal hernia. It kept getting bigger, and I kept wishing it to go away. I knew intellectually as a surgeon that eventually this would have to be surgically repaired, but I kept putting off the operation and delaying the obvious and only logical medical choice. My wife is a pediatric nurse and worked then in that capacity. Finally she reached her tolerance limit with my irrational fear of surgery for our son. As she always takes care of all of us, she told me calmly that she and our pediatrician had scheduled the operation. I was a wreck; I imagined him not surviving the simple operation and other complications only a surgeon could conceive. Even though I've operated on thousands of people, and they didn't die, the irrational fear was fixed in my mind, even as a surgeon, that something might happen.

Of course Josh had the operation and did fine. It was a non-event, and that was the end of it. This is the usual story. People have surgery every day. And for the patients who do have problems, we can generally trace back a story. Unless you're one of those people who have such unbelievable risk factors that they undertake an operation that is a desperation decision, the statistics clearly show that in almost all cases, you will do fine. Further, if your mind and body are prepared correctly—and you *will* be prepared if you follow my little plan—your surgery and outcome have much greater potential to be a beautiful event!

Pain and sleep dysfunction are the same. We become anxious even at the thought of pain or not being able to sleep, imagine it becoming worse, imagine that it will not go away or be out of our control, and the situation worsens. My father used to say that anger and fear are wasted emotions. What he meant by this was we spend a lot of time utilizing energy to deal with stresses in an abnormal way.

Logically we understand this is irrational, but our minds and thoughts are powerful and can easily overwhelm us until we realize that we are in control and can change them to suit our needs and desires. This is the magic of medical meditation.

2. Why are we afraid of surgery? Why do we take medications and drugs?

As I said above, we're all afraid of dying—it's natural, it's self-protective, and it's healthy. But let me tell you, you're not going to die in surgery. The statistics are way in your favor. Sure, people die every day, from heart attacks, cancer, car accidents, plane crashes, and yes, on rare occasions people die in the operating room. It's just their time. But I can pretty much tell you that dying is not something you need to worry about if you're relatively healthy and this is an elective operation, or you're reading this book. Even the sickest patients with many medical problems live through their operations. That doesn't mean that things can't go wrong, and of course you worry about that. But you can take steps to keep that from happening. Keeping yourself calm and healthy and being prepared are big steps. Being calm and healthy and making everyone else's life easier by being so also increases your chances of breezing through the day.

Learn to differentiate between the two types of fear that you are experiencing.

1. Realistic or rational fear

2. Emotional or panicking fear

Realistic fear is that something won't go completely right. The doctor was having a bad day and operates on the wrong extremity, or someone gives you a medicine you are allergic to. These are realistic fears and anxieties. Obviously things happen, but if you're calm and help everyone else through the day, likely everything will go according to plan. Statistics bear this out; most operations are successes, and many years of data and training for all involved are the reason we know this to be true. I had one patient years ago who drew her entire fracture as well as our plan for the operation on the cast so that when I removed it, I knew what was happening. I was amused and also quite relieved to know we were working together to get her better, and she did! I had another patient who marked in magic marker "cut here" to remind me of exactly where to work—the operating room staff had a great time ribbing me about that one! Although the patient was joking and knew that I knew what I was doing, it made us all laugh and feel more comfortable, and frankly it made me 100 percent sure I was with the right person at the right time and on the correct arm.

Irrational fear is when our minds get carried away. We begin to actually create scenarios of things going awry instead of going as planned. We think about stories we've heard, things we've read, and all the media hype that tells us everything that can possibly go wrong in this world. When our minds start running in these directions, they begin creating unrealistic fears and anxieties. If you've never had a heart attack, have no family history of heart disease, and have a healthy heart with healthy EKGs, worrying about having a heart attack from surgery is probably something you need not do. My friend Marty Rossman in his book *The Worry Solution* gives some great coping concepts for this. What it really comes down to is simply this: Visualize yourself as happy, healthy, and relaxed, visualize the day as going on as it should, and you will be fine and the day will go well, just as planned, and frankly, from a medical point of view, as expected.

The more you practice this visualization, the easier it is to recreate it, so when the day comes, you'll begin listening to the audio and your mind will automatically go to that happy, healthy, and relaxed state. You will be busy focusing on healing, feeling wonderful, and your life being exactly as it is supposed to be, and not a second thought to any of these anxieties will be there. If they do creep in, you will have the tools to gently brush them away.

Remember that you control your mind, and your mind controls your body—this book is about teaching you how.

CHAPTER 17

We All Want Control

Although it would be nice, you cannot be your own surgeon. It has been stated that the doctor who treats himself has a fool for a physician. I cannot do my own operations, but I can take care of myself medically, and using medical meditation and self-hypnosis techniques, I can prevent and repair illnesses and disease as well as injuries.

So the fact is, while you cannot train yourself to do your own operation or even to assist in surgery, you can maintain control and make a real difference in the outcomes.

The same holds true for dealing with pain and stress. Indeed there are times when something is needed to "take the edge off." Sometimes medications are necessary, but there are many choices, and which is safe for you? Further, how much do you need? The question to ask is how the medication or other pain-relief techniques can be most effective while using the lowest amount necessary of addictive medication. The answers are not as elusive or exotic as they may seem. Taking care of you and being in charge of your healing is a lot easier than we are led to believe. That is because there is big money to be made in convincing us all that we need the drugs or that we need to be taken care of!

Nurse Sally

Talk about taking charge of your healing—medical professionals are the toughest at each extreme! Sally was an operating room nurse I worked with who wanted to do just that: be in charge when I operated on her carpal tunnel. She wanted to assist in the operation and watch closely to be sure I did everything just right! She was a good friend, and we had worked together for many years. She trusted me as I did her. She really wanted to be part of her surgery and healing. I was young in my career and went for it. We allowed her to scrub in for her own procedure and set her up to hold her own retractors with the free hand. We allowed her to remain in a relaxed state and positioned her so that she could see everything. All went just right until I made the incision. It seems human nature dictates for most of us; seeing a stranger's insides is not the same as watching your own operation. Sally passed out as soon as we started. Once she knew she had control, she emotionally delegated this to me; she had helped get it started and promptly fell into a blissful, deep sleep. She did fine and actually needed less anesthesia as well as less medication postoperatively—we both learned something that day.

Sally taught me that we need to participate from the inside out, not the outside in. Simply doing a mechanical operation or prescribing a pill is not what the healing is about. Preparing your body and your mind to heal even before the process starts is what you are about to learn. You will prepare the body to heal and let the surgeon put things back in the right alignment to allow your body to heal them just as medicine opens a gate to your body's hormones to do the real job of healing or pain relief. You are the guide, overseeing the project from within. You will give your doc the sense and image of your healing by your calmness, or at least lack of complete panic, long before the operation begins. Leave the technical details to your surgeon. After the surgery, your medical meditation and self-hypnosis allow you to literally manifest the mental imagery, the picture of yourself as happy, healthy, and relaxed. What we have come to know is, when you imprint that picture of you healed on your subconscious mind, it has no choice but to manifest as reality by simply secreting the correct hormones and healing changes in your body...even before the operation begins. You control the process and the outcome simply by relaxing.

With pain and medication, it is the same thing. Your body secretes its own endogenous morphine, the most powerful pain reliever known to man/womankind. When you relax and see yourself healing, when you divert your attention to happy visions and feeling good, it adds endorphins and enkephalins, the feel-good hormones, and suddenly you begin to feel better, and you do not need the external stimulus, the pill, to produce the effect. Your body learns how to do it for you because it knows how to please you, to give you what you want!

Perhaps initially you will want and need some help, some medication, splints, braces, therapy, and this is fine. The mind works along with whatever you give it. Eventually you reach a level of confidence that allows you to use less and less additional medicine or treatment, and the body handles the discomfort on its own; without your even consciously thinking about it, it begins to heal you...because your mind knows you want to feel good.

CHAPTER 18

Surgery Has Gotten a Bad Name

It's scary, thinking about someone taking a knife, cutting you open, and then sewing you back together with string, and this fear is healthy. In many cases this fear is based on stories we have read or heard, still envisioning pictures of surgery in the 1800s in primitive operating rooms where many people did die. There were no antibiotics, and there was no anesthesia. Indeed it was a very risky proposition.

Others are haunted by an earlier family or childhood misadventure in the emergency room, hospital, or even with surgery. Perhaps you had a bad cut or broken bone as a child, and a well-meaning staff member held or strapped you down while treatment was rendered, leaving memories of a very scary event and a lingering mistrust and apprehension about all doctors and medical encounters. This was a not uncommon practice years ago. Or perhaps a relative or someone you knew had an operation, and you heard the story time and time again about the "catastrophe that occurred in the hospital, resulting in the loss of dear Aunt

Tillie." You don't know or actually remember any details, and who knows what really happened; she may have been 103, but no matter, the story stuck, and the fear lingered.

Please don't misunderstand, I agree with appropriate fear; surgery is not something we should seek out. I've in fact written three books telling patients that surgery should be a last resort. It is something that you should do if you have tried all conservative avenues and nothing else will help you. Sometimes the decision is easy; you have a life-threatening illness or a cancer that must be operated on to ensure that you will optimize your chances that it will be gone for good or a badly broken bone which is too malaligned to heal properly. These decisions are no-brainers, and whether the operation is completely successful or not, you have no choice. Fortunately these are the exceptional cases; most operations are by choice and at times, they end up being choices we regret. So you need to think carefully before you go to the operating room or decide to take narcotics or mind-altering medication. Learn to trust your own judgment and more importantly, learn other ways to heal and take care of yourself which allow you choices, rather than simply following the advice of one medical professional who may not have thought of other options than the medications or surgery. There are always choices, and you may choose surgery or the drugs, but be informed and certain of your choice and then you can be bold. In this way fear of the unknown lessens because you have confidence in your decisions and also you have choices that you have created by simply learning these techniques. Having confidence in your decision is key to full faith and belief in the process, whatever you choose to do.

Once you fulfill these criteria, you can let go and remember that you can still have control, even if that control is to give exactly that over to someone you trust.

A side note:

It is my personal and medical experience that many times surgery as well as medications can be avoided if one learns about the optional treatments for many medical problems. The fact is that most people do not know how to heal themselves. Explore alternatives; it is pretty easy today to do a thirty-minute internet search and see what medically rational alternative treatments exist for your problem. Remember, medical recommendations change quite often. Just last year the *Journal of the American Medical Association* came out with articles recommending a stomach-stapling operation as the first line of recommended treatment for obesity—even before trying dieting and exercise. Unbelievably, this included adolescents as well!

Do you really think this is the best and safest option? Surgery has complications, and changing normal anatomy has long-term effects that cannot be reversed. Remember it is not the operation that heals you, but your body that heals itself after the operation. In many, if not most instances, when you get your mind quiet, you decide not to take the risk and have an operation, take the pills, or take drastic action. Instead you may well decide to give some alternatives a try first. Maintain control, this is rule number one. You control your mind, and your mind controls your body. Except in very few circumstances, the choice is yours and yours alone. When you realize you have this control, you also begin to realize you can control much more of this process we call healing than you ever imagined.

CHAPTER 19

There Are No Minor Operations or Drugs without Side Effects

I guide my practice of medicine values keeping in mind a simple mantra taught to me years ago—*for physicians and healers, medical problems and diagnoses may be referred to as interesting, fascinating, intriguing, unique, and even puzzling. But when it comes to me, my family, and my patients, they are serious!*

In other words I always seriously consider everything that has to do with an operation, the writing of a medication, or a procedure before proceeding. Any operation, be it open-heart surgery or a simpler operation on your finger, requires meticulous attention - because it is being done to you and affects your well-being. How can we help assure this will happen? The answer is fairly simple; things go right when attitude, calmness, and focus on attention to detail all come together.

Any operation, be it a minor operation or major one, should have the same basic approach. First there is the thinking, the decision-making, and the preparation, as well as handling the anxiety that goes along with deciding to have an operation or take the pill in the first place. This process is daunting and is really something you really should take a little time to soul search.

Most operations are not emergencies. You have time and the ability to think about it; try alternatives and other options and be sure that you are making a decision that is good for you. Remember once you have an operation, you cannot take it back.

The same holds true for pain and medication choices. Pain from any cause, be it a broken bone, arthritis, or headache pain, is experienced differently by each of us. Learning to control or even lessen your pain, even to a minor degree, is a gift to yourself and allows healing to begin. Remember that your body produces its own endorphins and enkephalins, the feel-good hormones, as well as morphine, the most powerful pain reliever known to woman/mankind. Simply staying calm and learning how to focus your mind, along with a little practice, lets you learn to duplicate and enhance the effect of any medication - lessening, and even at times eliminating the need for that medicine. If nothing else, knowing you have some control over your pain and healing and limiting your dependence on the system or the pill is very important. You gain the power to decrease the control your pain and disease have over you and your body.

Here is a bit of information that you may not know:
It doesn't matter if you believe in meditation, prayer, hypnosis, magic, acupuncture, or faith healing. It does not matter if you are Catholic, Protestant, Buddhist, Jewish, Hindu, Muslim, or an atheist. What I'm teaching you here is simply a technique that you

can use to prepare yourself for healing an injury or operation. It is a technique that allows you to control pain, anxiety, sleep, and stress/anxiety. All you need to believe and understand is that there are certain proven miraculous capacities that all our bodies have, and when you relax, your body handles trauma, pain, and stress much better. Belief indeed is a powerful thing and will add to the effectiveness of what you are about to experience. If you simply follow the steps I outlined for you, your day of surgery or dealing with your injury or discomfort as well as the days to follow will be wonderful.

CHAPTER 20

Let's Begin Your Healing

By now you are beginning to see that your body has its own innate ability to heal and overcome disease.

Try this little exercise:

Did you know that by simply slowing your breathing to be less than eight breaths a minute, you drift into the alpha state, the entry to medical meditation that allows your blood pressure to lower and your heart rate to slow? You feel more relaxed and able to handle any insult to your body simply by breathing.

Close your eyes and begin counting ever so slowly backward from ten. Get in touch with your breathing, and just try to extend your "in" breath a little longer and your "out" breath even longer still. Slow down your breathing until you are sensing an easier and calmer pattern, and likely you will already be at less than eight breaths in a minute. You've just experienced the alpha state. Congratulations. Enjoy it for a few minutes.

If you are preparing for an upcoming procedure or operation, looking to gain better control of discomfort or to decrease dependence on medication, try this little exercise and then listen to the audio.

Audio #2: Begin your Medical Meditation - The Quick In-Out

CHAPTER 21

More Questions

What if after I decide to use medical meditation I panic, deciding I want regular medicine and anesthesia? The same question for decreasing or stopping my pain pills: What if I am in pain? What do I do? Can I go back to the old way?

Absolutely. It's OK to change your mind, even at the last minute. In fact I often use several methods of anesthesia, such as local anesthetic with sedation, to bring people to a very relaxed place, or sometimes I use a lighter general anesthetic along with hypnosis for my patients.

For the system it is all about costs and efficiency, and for my money, I want the choice! Don't skimp on making me and my patients comfortable.

With these techniques, at least you have a chance and much better options, since you already will know how to get relaxed and save *you* the trauma.

For all but the most extensive procedures, I will generally give patients options, choices.

Medical meditation and self-hypnosis allow you to have choices. This is in part because it helps your body do what is needed to experience your procedure calmly; you expect to feel better, to be happy and relaxed, and this allows everything to happen in a kinder, gentler way—surgery is less traumatic, medications work better, and your doctor becomes better because you calmly let her do what needs to be done.

The same holds true for medications in treating pain or anxiety or to help you sleep. Using these techniques will enhance the effect of any medication and let you decrease your dosage or use a less powerful medication that works equally well, often with fewer side effects or complications. Often an anti-inflammatory medication such as ibuprofen alternating with Tylenol along with meditation/self-relaxation gives equal or greater effectiveness to the narcotic opioid medicines. Plus, once you learn these techniques, you can teach your body to secrete its own morphine, duplicating the effect of the artificial one created by the medications, but with *zero* side effects. What a wonderful gift it is to give yourself relief and happiness by just closing your eyes for a few minutes!

How well does this work?

"I want this surgery to be a wonderful experience. Also I really do not like to be in pain—I am just not one of those people who says, 'I will just tough it out.' What do I do?"

Almost all my patients who have used these techniques tell me they've had wonderful experiences using medical meditation and self-hypnosis with surgery and for pain control. Even those who did no preparation and just listened to an audio before and during the procedure reported the same delight at the ease with which they handled the experiences. My practice is not alone in this experience. Dr. Elvira Lang, an invasive radiologist, uses similar techniques and reports the same outstanding success in helping people handle medical procedures in this relaxed and less drugged way.

Conversely those who have chosen not to learn or use these techniques often do not have as easy an experience, or they experience the unpleasant side effects of the drugs.

It is simple and predictable. My patients come to the operating room feeling relaxed and calm and have already started their own "anesthesia" before they even get to the operating suite. Not only do they require less medication and anesthetic, but they awaken feeling great. In fact the biggest complaint I hear in the recovery room is "I have to pee." I call my patients the evening after surgery, and more often than not they're still maintaining themselves, enjoying their own semi hypnotic trance, needing minimal if any medication, and though I generally write them a script just in case and they are free to use it, most do not or use very little. This is the beauty of self-control over your own body and healing.

I find the same experience in my patients with respect to medical meditation and medications. Many patients come to me who have long-standing nerve injuries and pain for which they have been taking opioid and mind-altering medications. Often, in fact, they find me looking for alternative ways to treat these injuries. They do not feel well on the medications, many are not enjoying life, and they do not like the way the medications make them feel. Their nights are dreamless, and they often tell me, "I want my life back." We incorporate these medical meditation techniques in their treatment, and most find they can decrease their medications, decrease their pain and discomfort, and use the medical meditation and self-hypnotic techniques to duplicate the effects of the medicines, which eventually decreases or eliminates the need for them. Plus they find that decreasing their sleep medications and sometimes antidepressant medicines allows them to return to their normal dreaming sleep and awareness of life; essentially, they return to joyful things in life and being themselves again.

I had a very interesting personal experience testing my own belief years ago. I had a large filling come out of a tooth. My dentist is also a close friend, and I went to see him in the office. He informed me that he would have to drill out what was left, do a root canal, and then refill the tooth. He told me this would be a deep drilling and could be quite uncomfortable. This doctor is a wonderful friend and a great teacher, and that day he had a resident with him. He also has a very keen sense of humor. He turned to his resident and said, "Dr. Fried uses hypnosis with his patients for surgery, so I am going to give him the choice." He then turned to me and said, "You can either have a shot of novocaine to numb this, or you can use self-hypnosis for this surgery!"

Well, even though I know hypnosis works, there was certainly some trepidation because this was my mouth. On the other hand, how could I not accept the challenge? I said, "Hypnosis, of course." But I forgot that dentists' offices are very busy.

He said, "Fine, I'll be back in five minutes and will do it." I placed myself into medical meditation, a hypnotic state, and numbed that side of my mouth. The procedure went flawlessly, and I enjoyed listening to them talk about how comfortable I looked (and I was) through the whole procedure. It was an enjoyable experience, and I never had a moment of discomfort, including afterward. I also knew that at any time if I had any discomfort,

I was free to ask for a shot to help. You always have the choice; that is the beauty of these techniques.

The same holds true for medications; you always have the choice to use them, but often you will find it is not necessary to take the pill if you relax and maintain control yourself. I sometimes play a game with myself if I have a strain or injury or headache. Instead of taking an anti-inflammatory pill, I simply put it in my pocket and roll it in my fingers. This reminds me that I have the option of a pill if I need one, and it allows me to relax and let the medical meditative state do the rest. I see myself feeling great and most often I do. The only problem with the technique is remembering to take the pill out of my pocket before it hits the laundry!

How good does it get?

One of the biggest challenges I faced over the years has not been the joy of teaching my patients how to use medical meditation and self-hypnosis to enjoy their procedures—quite the contrary. It's been in teaching the medical professionals that work with me its clinical effectiveness. Patients easily understand that positive thoughts and conversations make them feel better and help them stay positive in stressful situations. It's not entirely their fault, and once explained, almost all medical professionals embrace its power and effectiveness...in fact, many learn the techniques and use it with their own patients. Unfortunately there is very little training in medical school or residency for physicians about the power of their words and how what those in authority say can enhance or interfere with a great medical procedure or the effectiveness of a medication. This is even more the case when sedation has been given to the patient, since they are at a heightened state of acceptance to the words they hear.

CHAPTER 22

Placebo versus Nocebo

In the medical literature, for centuries, healers have used sugar pills, saline water injections, and many other substances to help people heal. These pills and injections have no real effect except that they make the patient believe they are being treated. And in fact, these placebo medications are still the standard of comparison in testing effectiveness of many new medicines developed today.

A recent study on the effectiveness of erectile dysfunction drug Cialis, when compared to a placebo, showed that both were equally effective in attaining erection. The takeaway—the patient's mind is the most powerful sexual organ, and when focused properly, it is much safer than a relatively dangerous pill.

There's an opposite to the placebo. It is called the nocebo; the nocebo effect is what happens when a medicine or a medical suggestion such as "This procedure is going to hurt" or "Your hair will always fall out with chemotherapy" is planted by a medical professional. In fact, many people who have chemo do not lose their hair, and many people do not have much discomfort after medical procedures or side effects from medications.

We as doctors and you as patients would be wise to remember to choose our words and those we discuss our medications, as well as procedures with, carefully. Staying positive is a wonderful way to go through a procedure, as well as live your life.

CHAPTER 23

The Dreaded Question

Whenever I begin working at a new hospital or with new staff, I enjoy teaching them the power of words and how suggestion is so important. I remind them that patients hear while under anesthesia, and there are those who at first do not believe me. Then they meet my patients and I ask them to follow my instructions, specifically requesting the recovery room, anesthesia, and operating room teams ask the right questions when my patients awaken from surgery. You see, when you use medical meditation, you expect to awaken feeling happy, healthy, and relaxed. Your expectation is that you will have little or no discomfort, and indeed that is usually the case. Don't misunderstand me; your body will always let you know if there is something going on that's dangerous or limb or life-threatening. But discomfort is just that, experienced at many different levels. So, you can guess what happens when you awaken from that beautiful, restful sleep and meditation, often assisted with mind-altering medications, and the first question you hear when you open your eyes is...

"Are you having any pain?"

Seriously, Doc, what do you expect to hear next? Even if you were feeling great, when redirected to focus on an area that's just been operated on, you will usually report some discomfort; even if you don't feel it, you will now be expecting it, so you search for any signs of it. So you say, "Why yes, I am having pain, discomfort, a twinge...thanks for focusing me on that." Then you are given medication, get nauseated, and have a lousy experience. Instead if we medical professionals simply ask, "How do you feel," guess what? Most of my patients tell me about the wonderful dream they had, where they went in that dream, and what an enjoyable day they were having. Let me tell you, that makes my day just as enjoyable! Sure, if they do have discomfort, they let me know, and we can address that, but in terms of what will take the edge off, not make them sick from overmedicating. Expect to feel happy, healthy, and relaxed, and that is exactly what you will experience. Note: If you are having surgery, talk to your surgeon and especially your anesthesiologist about this. Tell them you are a positive thinker, you practice relaxation, and would appreciate when you awaken being asked "How do you feel?" or "Is there anything we can get you?" They might chuckle, but hopefully they will go along with the program. If not, at least request that you can listen to a tape and keep your headphones on throughout the procedure and play these tapes or whatever you like that makes you happy... keep control of your world.

CHAPTER 24

Live independent of the good opinion of others.
—Dr. Herbert Maslow

Maslow has a simple answer for life in a better way. Everyone will give you their stories; everyone will tell you how *your* surgery is going to be experienced, what you are going to feel, and how you must act. Everyone has an opinion, from your family to friends to the surgeon and anesthesiologist as well as the nurses. These opinions are based on what we in medicine call circumstantial evidence, one case here and one there, limited experiences and experiential evidence. This is in contradistinction to solid, empirical medical evidence based on facts and well-thought-out and implemented medical studies. This is why we have peer-reviewed journals. I am a reviewer for the medical journal *HAND*, a well-respected hand surgery journal. When an article is submitted, we want it to be based on real clinical evidence, not circumstantial evidence. And guess what? The scientific evidence about surgeries across the board is well established; most people do just fine with surgery, and especially in advanced medical societies, almost all survive and have no long-term ill effects from their operations. So if you are having surgery, *let it go*. And certainly let go of everyone else's opinions. You and your experience are no one else's business. Place your own expectations in your mind. See the surgery as a healing, happy process or a process that simply needed to be done. Don't have an expectation of how you might feel. Expect you will feel great—happy and healthy—and that this will do wonderful things for you. Your expectation is generally what you receive. And don't worry about insulting other people or ignoring "the experts." You know you and your body better than anyone. You know how you tolerate things, the events of life, cuts, bruises, medications, and the like. If you are a person who screams in agony when you have your fingernails cut, then you may have a lower tolerance for discomfort than someone who pulls splinters out of himself or sews his own wounds shut when he cuts himself. Somewhere in the middle is where most lie. Begin to understand that you are in control. But remember that your operation or your medical condition is being handled by experts, and the nice thing about this situation is that if you do experience discomfort, all you need to do is ask and this can be made to feel better...from anxiety before the operation to making you comfortable in the recovery room. So you have your meditation, your preparedness, and your medical team all on your side to meet your every need. Last time you had that you were still in diapers!

CHAPTER 25

A Patient Story

You may wonder how powerful the mind can be in overcoming words said around you—the reality is, pretty darned powerful. Obviously none of us will likely experience the challenge Suzie, one of my patients, did, but what I learned from this extraordinary lady is that taking a little time and using meditation to block out the distractions surrounding us can often make dealing with less-than-pleasant situations a lot easier.

After training in our medical meditation and self-hypnosis program, Suzie had a terrifying incident but one that turned out wonderfully thanks to her ability to control her own physiology through medical meditation and self-hypnosis. She was in a very bad car accident and had injuries so severe that they initially called a helicopter to transport her to the hospital; they weren't certain she was going to make it. In fact, they sent back the helicopter believing there was nothing that could be done.

She had significant bleeding, and though the situation was quite hectic, her first inclination was to block out all the chaos. Somehow she managed to keep her head together enough to calm herself down. When she used these techniques, the meditative state brought her heart rate and basic metabolic levels down so low that the bleeding stopped, and she stopped hemorrhaging, saving her own life! She was taken by ambulance to the hospital where the medical team feared she would be pronounced dead. But her subconscious had other ideas. Upon arrival at the hospital, when she heard the doctors talking, she knew subconsciously she was in a place that could help her.

Suzie awakened, began to bleed again, and to everyone's surprise, they found that Suzie was very much alive. The medical team was able to perform the appropriate procedures to save her, and she ultimately recovered and did very, very well. She is alive, well, and normal today thanks to her ability to control her own physiology.

Now, in fairness to all of us, Suzie is one of our more advanced students with meditation, but she is a great example of how impressive simply letting go and believing in our innate abilities to control our healing really can be. Hers is not an extraordinary ability as much as a powerful belief in the process—she knows it works!

CHAPTER 26

What Do I Mean by Having Surgery and Healing Pain "The Easy Way?"

"Medical meditation and self-hypnosis themselves are simply fixed, focused states of attention, and be sure—when you are about to cut someone—you do have their attention! This can be used to everyone's benefit."
—Dr. Scott Fried, American Association for Surgery of the Hand Annual Meeting

I've spent the past quarter of a century operating on people and helping them get better with and without surgery. The above quote was from my introductory comments to a room full of surgeons at a national meeting. When you do this kind of work and you take the time to get to know your patients, their lives, why they have surgery, and most importantly, how they do after surgery, you learn a lot from them.

Eastern medicine has as its basis the philosophy that the body heals, and the less we can do to it to interfere with that the better. The same holds true for surgery and medications. Surgery is not a natural event but rather an assault on your body. Yes, it is done in the name of healing, but nonetheless it is traumatic. Medications are not natural either but artificially stimulate your body to secrete the real healing substances.

So when I say the easy way, I simply mean that when you are prepared in the proper manner, mentally and physically, and your biological systems are relaxed and ready, the process goes more smoothly, much like anything else in life.

These are not just techniques for people who are "naturals" in meditation, like monks who sit in and melt snow at the top of the mountain. This is for you and me, everyday people. We have been brainwashed by the medical industry to think we can't take care of ourselves. We have been programmed to think that we are helpless and that only the almighty institution or physician can make us feel better. Your mind is more powerful than any medication we can get you. In fact, by using these techniques you can gift yourself anesthesia, muscle relaxation, and the ability to limit discomfort - any time you want.

CHAPTER 27

Four Simple Steps to Master the Opioid Alternative

Below are a few simple guidelines, and if you follow them, your day of surgery or dealing with your pain or sleep will be a little more like a nice walk in the park.

Prepare, Prepare, Prepare!

Step Number 1: Final Decisions

Get ready for your surgery. First and foremost, decide if you should have it; if your situation is limb or life-threatening, and if time is of the essence—go for it! The same holds true for medications.

If, on the other hand, your life is not in imminent danger, consider part of your preparation a true soul search. You and you alone will live with whatever decision you make.

Learn all you can about what you have, why you have it, and what the alternative options are. Seek out opinions to allow you to decide what feels right to you. Perhaps you think therapy or acupuncture or some other medical treatment that is less invasive might help; why not give it a try? Check with the person who specializes in that therapy or treatment, not necessarily a surgeon. Remember, although we as surgeons make our best decisions based on our training (and most are highly ethical and moral people), surgeons are optimally trained and also get paid to cut people. So like it or not, there is an incentive bias there, as with each specialist, to believe they have the ultimate solution. Pain doctors are the same situation. They have extensive training and knowledge in powerful and often addictive/mind-altering medications as well as spinal nerve block, injections, and implant procedures. This is their training and what they are likely to use, so again, it is not malicious, but these too have substantial possible complications and consequences.

Conversely, physical and occupational therapists, massage therapists, acupuncturists, and homeopathic and chiropractic medical professionals are trained to believe that they can cure you. The complications are less severe, and often the results are quite effective, equal to successful surgery. This does not mean that no one should have surgery or take medications; it just means that these options might be considered, but sometimes those trained in alternative healing also let their bias stand in the way of getting surgery or using medications. It is not necessarily their training to go that route, so they may hold back that recommendation because that was how they were trained.

Getting the picture? Each medical professional is trained with a certain mindset, and therefore ultimately the best person to decide your path is you.

Try to fully understand and search out what other treatment options might help your situation. Maybe even let time heal it. This works for a large percentage of back pain patients. Are you in a rush or have you no choice?

In other cases you might consider if this potential operation is one that's simply saving you some personal work or a challenge you do not want to face? For instance some people have stomach-stapling operations to help them lose weight. And yes, there are certainly people who need this operation in that their weight gain is due to medical issues beyond their control, but they are the exceptions, not the rule. There are complications with these procedures, as with any operation, so why not try alternatives first?

Fact: The body loses weight if it eats fewer calories. It's that simple. Yes, it is more demanding, but certainly there are few complications caused by eating less, not always so for abdominal surgery. Wayne Dyer points out in one of his books, "It takes a lot more work to prepare food, serve it, chew it, swallow it, and digest the food...as compared to just not eating it." Quite logical, and the yield in the latter is fewer calories going in! The man makes a good point.

Or take for example prostate surgery. Until recently, prostate biopsy and surgery were done in many patients who had blood tests showing there may be possible prostate cancer. This is a very slow-growing malignancy and in many cases can be observed rather than aggressively treated. Many patients have difficult complications such as scarring in the area, pain, sexual dysfunction, and painful constriction of their urethra, and studies show significant depression resulting from these surgical treatments. In fact a recent study showed that patients who chose observation and regular checks for their prostate cancer did essentially equally well with the conservative treatment as with surgery, and now the recommendation is to discuss the options with your doctor because outcomes are nearly identical and the side effects are substantially less without surgery. Further, a number of patients who chose surgery had a higher rate of depression and many required antidepressant medications, with all their added side effects, as compared to almost none in the group who chose not to have surgery. Currently in many patients over sixty-five, the recommendation for prostate problems including cancer becomes watchful waiting.

Of course each case is individual, and there are many factors that go into what is right for each patient. But more than one opinion is a very good idea before rushing into many of these surgeries. This doesn't hurt the outcome and might save you a lot of time and discomfort. Know your options.

I recommend careful consideration of everyone's own case, and to be clear, many people absolutely do need surgery, and if you and your doc agree on that, you should proceed with a clear conscience. This is where these techniques are of great value.

The same holds true for painful conditions. Often there are excellent treatments that allow you other options than medications or treatments that decrease the discomfort enough that you do not need opioid and heavily sedating or mind-altering medications. This is exactly what this book is about, seeking alternatives and knowing options, so that if you do decide to have surgery or begin medications which have real side effects, you know you have considered other options; then relaxation and meditation will make these more invasive treatments easier and lessen the need for extended and or excessive opioid use.

Bottom line:

Reactive Living—if you live in a reactive state, reacting to what people tell you rather than your gut instinct, which is usually fear of surgery or fear of pain, then it is very difficult to relax. Your body's natural impulses are good; they protect you. Trust these intuitions instead of the scary scenario of a medical society that imposes medical treatment dogmas on patients rather than including them in the decision making. If you remain in charge, you will remain calm.

Trust your mind, trust your body, and trust yourself. Your body has a wonderful innate capacity to heal and innate wisdom to know what is best for you.

Write it down! Write down your thoughts, your plans, and your options. Look at your thoughts and keep them on one page. This is something that is personal, just for you, to help in decision making. When you write things down you see them much more clearly.

Questions might be:

- How bad do I really feel; how much do I hurt? Why might I be experiencing this?

- What are my other options?

- If I have surgery or take opioid medications, what are the chances they will help cure me?

- What are the complications and risks?

- What are the benefits, and what will the long-term outcome look like? What else might I do or try before going down this path?

- Am I certain I want to or need to do this, or at least as certain as I can be?

Though these questions are for you alone, if you cannot come to conclusions or need to ask others their opinions, try to ask those you truly trust and perhaps other experts in the field who have various viewpoints, as we discussed above. Perhaps you are lucky enough to have a family doc or ob-gyn who knows you well as a person. Try to avoid simply asking random friends and even family, other than for support, since they all have opinions and personal stories, but not always the factual knowledge to help with a best decision. That is not to say abandon those you love and who care about you; they may well offer support emotionally and life insights but try to find solid insight from factual sources to make your ultimate decision. And trust your inner being most.

If you can answer these questions comfortably and know in your heart that the decision is right to go ahead with surgery or the medications, then you will be able to use the tools below to your best advantage.

If on the other hand you decide not to have surgery or use the opioids, what is below will help you achieve that as well. And remember, you can always change your mind if the path you have chosen is not working out.

Step Number 2: Do It Your Way

Once you've decided to have surgery or to use a medication, be comfortable that you are still in charge of what goes on in your mind. But for God's sake, once you've made the decision, let go— release control to your doctor and let it happen. As soon as you begin to see yourself healed, it will begin to manifest. You know what's healthy for you, and you know that you have made a good and informed decision to proceed with this operation.

A wonderful study was done by an orthopedic surgeon, Bruce Mosley, who was the team physician for the Houston Rockets. He suspected that a very common knee operation might not be quite as good at healing people as believed. In fact he thought that possibly the operation was a sham, and it was the expectation of surgery helping that healed patients rather than the actual procedure. He devised and carried out a study where he divided his patients into three groups. The operation is called a debridement, and it is done with an arthroscope, a small telescope that lets us look into the knee. Then a separate instrument called a shaver is inserted, and this reams out the inflamed tissue called synovitis and the degenerated cartilage in the knee, the stuff arthritis is made of. The debridement removes the bad tissue with the theory that this treats arthritis.

Preoperatively he told each of the patients in the three groups the truth: that some of them were going to get a full operation, the arthroscope in the knee, shaving out the arthritis, and washing out with irrigation anything else harmful. The second group would get the arthroscope put in the knee joint and the washing out. The third group would simply have a nick made in the skin and nothing more—no arthroscope, no washing out or shaving out the arthritis, no operation at all.

Now mind you, all of them knew that they might have any of the three operations. One in fact was not an operation at all. When the results were compiled, to the surprise of the surgical community, but not to Mosley, simply the expectation that they would feel better after the operation resulted in outstanding results in relief in all three groups! That is right, equal relief and healing was achieved no matter what was done. Mosley proved that this operation was a sham procedure and further that it was the expectation of a wonderful outcome that created the result—the patients' minds, not the surgery!

Never underestimate the power of your mind.

Again, medications and expected results from these are the same. Study after study shows the effectiveness of placebos with sham medications having almost equal or better effectiveness than the actual drugs. This is your mind and your physiology producing the desired results because you create that expectation and subsequently that manifests in your physiology.

How are you personally going to prepare for the surgery? Is your body in the best shape for the operation? Are you at the right weight? Is your diet right, one that is optimal for you healing? If you're a smoker, have you cut down so that you will breathe more easily upon awakening and during the surgery?

Begin to think about how you would like to meditate that day. What would you like to listen to? How are you going to listen, do you have a phone and audio player that you can take to the operating room? What are you going to listen with, a headset or other device? I use a meditation mask with my patients which has audio speakers in it that we developed. It works great and allows patients to completely tune out or open the "view" window and see what is going on. What is important is that you begin

the planning and let your surgeon as well as the anesthesiologist
know you plan to use an audio relaxation tape. Most are open
to this and many welcome it. But it's best to ask.

My patients begin listening as soon as they arrive at the hospital, so they are relaxed the whole time. This is very helpful in
the preoperative area while you are waiting. It helps the time go
by and prepares your mind for a great day.

Begin seeing yourself as happy, healthy, and relaxed. Begin
eating as if you are already using the optimal diet to regenerate and repair. Begin your post-op therapy by conditioning and
stretching your body, whichever parts you can, before you ever
reach the operating room. Today you begin healing, not only from
your operation but for your life.

Step Number 3: You Are the Boss of You

When they were very young, on occasions when they became
frustrated, upset, or angry (yes, some of those times were indeed
my doing), I would tell our children that they could control their
emotions and the world around them. Although they were little,
and still not quite grasping the entire concept, they were often
open to this suggestion. I explained that they had power they
did not even know they had. Milton Erickson, the great psychiatrist and hypnotherapist, used to tell his patients that they knew
things they didn't even know they knew. What he meant by this
was that our subconscious mind understands what we and our
bodies need, and it knows how to make it happen. In fact that
is its job, to take care of us and secrete the correct hormones to
make healing and health happen. All we really need to do is just
get out of its way.

The same held true for our children. I would ask them, "Who is the boss of you?"

Initially they would say, "You are, Dad," or more often, of course, "Mom! She's the boss of all of us." Although the temptation was to agree with them on the latter statement, I would continue to ask them until they understood the answer.

Finally I would simply say: "Kids, you are the boss of you."

It did take a while for that to sink in, especially when we told them they could not have more candy or had to go to bed. As they got older, they argued that we still bossed them around. But the message was really clear, at least to me—you cannot make anyone do anything they do not want to, and each of us is clearly in control of our own mind and body. If you don't believe me, try to get a toddler who is not potty-trained to go on the toilet. You had better be prepared for a little "I am in control" pushback before it happens. What kid wants to get up and stop playing if they have to pee or poop when they can just do it in the diaper and deal with letting someone else clean it up later?

You see, we are all in charge, completely, of every decision we make. What you eat, how you care for your body, and whether you have this operation or take that pill are completely in your control. Yes, there are circumstances where emergencies happen, but it's not likely you're reading this book to prepare for an emergency. Hopefully if you do have an emergency in the future, you will still understand that you should maintain control of you and your body as best you can because this will still be the healthiest thing for you. In any case, since we are talking about electing to have an operation or take a medication, in this situation, you are the boss!

So why is this control so important? It's the gremlins!

Many years ago, when I was early in my training, I learned a great lesson from a very smart surgeon. He gathered us all around him and told us that we only had one job as medical students, to protect the patients, from the minute they walked in the hospital until they left, from the gremlins. It seemed an odd statement from a very well-respected surgeon, but then he explained.

The gremlins are the people and details in the course of a day that can make an easy stay a bit more challenging, or conversely, a lot more pleasant, if they are kept at bay. It may be the person who draws your blood before the operation or the one who interviews you for the hospital and tells you about all the possible problems you might face and possible complications that could happen, or the nurse who forgets to put up the guardrail on your bed. Perhaps it is a well-meaning doctor who wants to prescribe medication or a procedure that may help you, but feels it is incumbent on them to detail every possible outcome again, even though you have been well informed, instead of reassuring you .

Of course these scenarios people talk about are all far-fetched events that very rarely happen, and I am not suggesting you worry. Quite the opposite, I am preparing you for the fact that if you prepare yourself and let the professionals taking care of you do their job while you relax, it is much more likely that everyone will have a more positive experience. Your calmness will comfort and relax the people helping you, and they will do better for you.

You need to guard yourself from any negative influence in staying positive, not simply believing but knowing that the choices you have made were with the best information you could obtain and in keeping with your inner compass. Yes, of course, you need to hear and be aware of possible complications, but that should all be behind you well before you're in the final preparations for the operation. Hear them once, weigh them, and then put them aside and in the place they belong; you've already made an informed decision.

Do not let anyone distract you from your ultimate goal. Your goal is to be better and to start getting better before the process even begins. Let the family member, friend, or trusted professional take care of everything else that goes on around you while you focus your mind completely on happiness, health, and healing.

I cannot say this enough times. Do not let anyone but you control your thinking and healing thoughts. Anything but positive influences must be avoided if at all possible. You have made a decision, and it is yours and yours alone to make. Once you have, eliminate any naysayers. Don't even speak to people who are going to give you anything except positive reinforcement. Once the decision has been made and you have consulted with those you trust and feel the decision's right, move away from anything but positive influences. Do not be distracted or dissuaded from your goal.

One caveat: You may at some point in the preparation process change your mind. Know that at any time, if you decide you should not have this operation, that is OK. This is not about bravado. As happens in life, things change; you are allowed to change your mind. You are allowed to delay the operation for any reason. Perhaps you're feeling better; yes, this is possible. Sometimes when you begin to visualize your healing, when you begin treating your body as if it has healed before the operation, you do begin to get better, and healing occurs. I've seen this many times. So if you feel better and you think the problem is going away, don't be afraid to hold off. As long as it's not a life-threatening problem, consider waiting a bit if the healing is occurring and you feel it.

One thing to remember about surgeries—once you have them, you can't take them back.

The same thing often happens with medications. Early on, when we started using meditation and relaxation with patients to help them sleep and decrease their pain, many of them came to me and told me that other things were happening in their body. They noted their blood pressure was lower, or their cholesterol levels were coming back at lower numbers than previously. I recall a specific patient, Janet, who came to me and said, "Hey Doc, I am going to stop my blood pressure and cholesterol medication."

I knew her well, and in fact she's not a person that messes around; if she says she's going to do something she does. I told her, "Wait a minute, I'm an orthopedic surgeon; I'm not cardiologist or family doctor. Before you just stop taking your medication, please check with your doctor."

Janet came to me the following week and told me that her doctor said she should continue these medications; she asked why, and he said, "Because I take them!" She said that was not good enough but did come to a compromise that she'd go another month with a reduced dose and see if her numbers continued to get better. Well, they did, and she ultimately was able to stop her medications. Later a study proved what Janet intuitively knew; meditation and relaxation along with a little exercise and red yeast rice has equal benefit for many to the cholesterol-lowering medication she was taking. I already knew from the work of Dr. Herbert Benson that lowering blood pressure was a predictable outcome from meditation and self-hypnosis. Janet simply validated that science!

Step Number 4: Insight and Intuition—Trusting Your Inner Knowing.

Each of us has knowledge and insights we're not even aware of that help us relax and heal. Innately we each understand things that we seemingly have no reason to, but yet we do. Some call this intuition; others chalk it up to memories or perhaps past lives lived, I sometimes call it your inner knowing. This is not a matter of IQ or superior intelligence; it is basic instinct. In fact it is often hindered by our intelligence or our thinking that we know better than what our body is telling us, since I know many very intelligent people who care for themselves very poorly, including, perhaps especially, physicians!

My great friend Dr. Marty Rossman, a well-known authority on imagery and its use in analysis, calls this insight by a name: "our inner adviser." In fact using meditation and relaxation techniques with imagery allows you to better get in touch with this inner adviser of yours. I personally have had a few, and one was our dog Chuckie, who clearly was a wizard. He was calming, and his eyes showed you the wisdom of being unconditionally calm and loving. He was a soothing soul and brought great comfort to our family when life got hectic.

To get in touch with your inner adviser is relatively simple. You simply use the techniques you are learning here to place yourself in a very quiet, calm state, your medical meditation and self-hypnosis—find a quiet place that feels safe and open and comforting to you, and then let your mind drift to begin thinking about someone or something who's kind, caring, and wise. Perhaps you might know or admire someone you consider very wise and knowledgeable. Whatever image comes to your mind, as long as it is caring, loving, and you feel safe with this adviser, simply accept it. You might even begin to dialogue with this adviser and ask questions or share concerns. This dialogue may be actual words or occur in other ways such as a feeling, a comfortable silence, or perhaps a smile. It is simply a communication with your deep subconscious, your inner mind, and inner knowing. Often answers come to us concerning problems, challenges, fears, and struggles, offering ways to heal and feel. You might consider trying this and see what images come to you. It's always nice to have a friend going through the process with you, even if it's an imaginary one. It certainly worked for many of us as children, didn't it?

Remember this—the natural tendency of your body is to heal. In fact our body heals with no effort from our conscious mind at all because that is what your subconscious mind does—it takes care of you. And it does it miraculously and efficiently. The key is getting out of its way. Surgery and medications temporarily and at times necessarily get in its way, and you must heal after surgery and rid your body of the side effects of medications and or anesthesia. So when you are relaxed and your consciousness sees yourself as happy and healthy and already healed, your subconscious mind knows no difference between fantasy and reality, so it begins healing, almost ignoring and bypassing the insults. That is not to say it interferes with what surgery's meant to do; it just takes what your surgeon has done and makes it even better. Remember we as surgeons simply line things up and the body does the rest!

There are countless studies showing that using meditation and self-hypnosis enhances your immune system. It sends healing cells such as lymphocytes to fight infection, as well as fibroblasts which repair injured tissues to the area in need, speeds healing of wounds, and optimizes all the natural functions of our body and its systems. It also allows us to reset our thermostat, our perception of pain and discomfort. This is why we can actually do surgery, dental work, injections, and full operations without any anesthesia. Your body has its own anesthesia and knows how to use it. In fact it allows us to safely ignore discomfort, although if it is a discomfort or pain that is limb or life-threatening, your subconscious will always allow that to come through and protect you.

Okay, you are ready for a full healing session so please listen to Audio #3:
A Healing Session - Healing Sand

CHAPTER 28

Questions about the Doomsday World

I know I should ignore all the naysayers and the people who tell me it's going to be horrible, but I just can't help feeling it's going to be a stressful experience. Am I the only one who is afraid of surgery?

No, it's not you. This society is a marketing and propaganda, as well as hypnotic suggestibility, machine. Every day you are bombarded with messages.

Just turn on the television at night and see how many commercials there are for sleep, anxiety, and depression medications. You may notice that they always come on right after the doomsday sensationalizing news! Flip through any magazine and see how many articles there are about medicines, surgeries, and cosmetic surgeries to change you and your world and your life, making us all feel that we can never live up to the plastic society they pretend is reality, simply to sell products. That's what sells! News is big business, mind manipulation...and the worse it sounds and the more attention-grabbing, the better. People make a living on your fears, anxieties, and deep-rooted desire to be happy. You're taught to worry about screenings and diagnostic tests, to be sure that you get on cholesterol-lowering medication, and to avoid high blood pressure. Sure, good medicine is great, and if you see your doctor, she will likely make sure you are taken care of, specifically for the things that apply to you. But everyone is not sick; most are well until they are stressed out enough.

I bet you don't see any commercials saying, "Learn meditation, and to relax, do a little exercise and take care of yourself, and guess what? You won't need medications or the operations." Why? Because there is no money in that for the system; in fact it loses the big businesses millions of dollars when people relax a little and take care of themselves.

The bottom line is—sure you're scared because that's what's created. The industry wants you to be scared and then pay them to take care of you.

When you feel scared or overwhelmed, and you feel like this is getting to you, just put on the audio and practice these techniques. You'll see how quickly these fears fade away, and you'll awaken calm and relaxed, feeling more in control. The more you practice this, the better it gets.

Self-help author Napoleon Hill in the 1930s told a wonderful story about his son who was born with no ears. Medicine in the early 1900s was not sophisticated, and he was told by doctors that his son would never hear. But Hill was a man who believed. He believed in himself and the fact that anything he put his mind to he could achieve. He taught millions of people the secrets of growing rich—riches in life as well as dollars. And he set himself on the mission to allow his son to hear, despite what he had been told by the doctors. When his son was very young, he would walk around him clapping and clapping behind him, until one day he actually got a response. He ultimately found a doctor with a similar mindset, and what they came to understand was that the bones of the child's skull actually transmitted sound, much like the bones of the inner ear. Even in the early part of the last century, they were ultimately able to fashion a crude device that was an early hearing aid, and ultimately his son gained almost 80 percent normal hearing; he went on to speak and live a normal life. This was due partly to Hill's belief that he could succeed and his ignoring all the naysayers and the doctors who told him that there was nothing that could be done.

It never fails to astound me that people accept that surgery will be an unpleasant, uncomfortable, and dismal experience or a well-meaning medical professional's statement that "Nothing more can be done" or "You will always have pain or suffer as you do." These patients understandably become despondent, dependent on drugs, and some even suicidal. In fact I find for my patients it's the opposite. As a subspecialist I have the privilege of meeting so many of these patients, and more often than not there is a lot that can be done. Many go on to heal, avoid further surgeries, and rid themselves of their dependence on medications.

It becomes an exciting (and yes, sometimes challenging) time but generally the beginning of a healing. The same holds true for those with long-standing pain and medication dependence; once they understand the control they have over their own bodies and lives, they find a path that allows them to move ahead with healing themselves. The key is in expectation and belief that you can be in control of your world, no matter what is going on around you, from within yourself.

I remember when my wife was pregnant with our first child. She and two of my colleagues' wives were pregnant as well. They were all in nursing, and we were all educated surgeons. We went to a class, and the first thing the woman teaching the class on natural childbirth said was, "If you end up having a C-section, you're a failure." All six of us stood up and left. This type of misinformation is clearly not only incorrect and ignorant but also destructive. Any woman who carries a child for nine months, no matter how she gets it out of her body, is a hero! If a C-section is what it takes to save my child's life and have her come out normal and healthy, then that is the way it should go. What I learned, even back then, was that the thoughts that are placed in our heads can be very dangerous, especially from those who have "perceived authority or knowledge." Luckily, as medical professionals, we had the understanding to walk out and find someone who allowed our wives to have a choice and be in control of their own bodies and lives.

There is nothing worse than feeling helpless in a situation. Control is something that we all want, but in reality, none of us ever gain it over anything except ourselves. But here is the trick. You are always in control of yourself and your inner world. No matter what goes on around you and what others might say or do, if you can remain calm and keep yourself in a relaxed state, everything will be all right. Once you understand that you can control your physiology and your actual thermostat of registering discomfort or creating your own anesthesia, you realize that not only can you have a pleasant operative experience, but you will! And your control also allows you to ask for and or use any of the medicines or treatments that are available as well, if *you* so choose. That is the difference; you are in control of your body and your world.

CHAPTER 29

Understanding the Medical System

When I talk to patients about surgery, medications, healing, and how the medical system works, I'm consistently amazed that most people have no idea that they are in control. In fact most people feel helpless to even take care of themselves. They've been programmed by our media and frankly by my colleagues and our society to "be taken care of."

I have a good friend who has at his disposal some of the best medical care in the world. He is a very wealthy man, with excellent connections in the medical community, and he can see any doctor he wants and attain any treatment, home device, or medication that he desires. He is very intelligent and very capable. He had some significant problems from an old injury to his neck. He tried everything, including medications, therapy (which actually made him worse), epidural injections in his spine, and multiple other various treatments. He was told that surgery would help, but that it of course could also paralyze him. We discussed this at various times, and I taught him medical meditation/self-hypnosis. The focus of self-hypnosis for him was to relax and to see healing options. We hadn't spoken for a few months when he called me. He told me that he had a realization while meditating that he could be in control of his healing. He changed the exercise routine that was given to him and his diet, took charge of his own healing, let go of the system controlling him - and he healed. He still has the same X-ray findings and ongoing pathology in his neck, but he has minimal symptoms and does not need to use a bag of ice on his neck every night, injections, or medications on a regular basis. Nor does he experience daily discomfort—all because he took charge of his own body and healing.

I hear so often from people that they haven't got time to take care of themselves—time to change the way they eat, to get enough sleep, or to exercise. In fact we have been told by society that if we sleep too much, we are lazy. We should try to work more, stress more, and be "more productive." Educational studies show that college athletes actually score better on tests than their peers, and many are better students. The fact is, keeping your body physically fit, be it regular exercise or at the level of NCAA athletes who spent twenty or more hours a week training, makes you more efficient and sharper in every way. These athletes' schedules give them much less time to study, sleep, and have fun, but they still perform extraordinarily well in college. Plus they look and feel great! So the excuse that there is no time to exercise and still be productive really doesn't hold up. The same holds true for meditation; a few minutes used to relax and focus make someone extraordinarily more productive.

When Einstein had a problem that was perplexing him, he played the violin, and this cleared his mind of the clutter that stood in the way of the answers he sought. It doesn't take being Einstein to see the benefit in taking a break, now, does it?

As to eating, it is very ceremonial. We eat as we do for a thousand different reasons. Some of this is cultural, some by developed tastes, and much of it out of habit. I myself was raised eating a very unhealthy diet. When in my residency in training I lived on fast foods, pasta, and bread. I also weighed thirty pounds more than I do now. I did not eat fish, and no one could convince me that I should. I went through a period when I was not feeling well, and I used self-hypnosis to program my mind to eat better, feel better, and be more energetic—and just like that, once my subconscious saw what I wanted, I changed my eating habits. It wasn't hard, in fact the process was enjoyable. I was in charge, and I was able to choose what I wanted to eat. I now eat fish, salads, chicken, and very little red meat and feel much better. I was not trying to lose weight but lost thirty pounds and got to my correct weight. I feel better, and I'm in charge. I see this time and time again when my patients choose to eat differently and feel better as well as heal better.

One of the things we need to know about surgery is that the more excess weight we have, the longer it takes for the anesthesia to get out of our system and our lungs to clear. The medications build up in fat, so losing a few pounds before surgery is greatly helpful. Also, excess weight makes healing from operations more difficult. In fact it makes breathing itself more difficult. Our body must work harder to support the extra weight in many ways. From an orthopedic standpoint, for example with knees, people can often delay or even avoid knee replacement surgery or back surgery if they lose even a little weight by decreasing the stress on the joints as well as the spine. And for people who do have surgery, excess weight is much harder on the implants and on the spine in the healing and long-term process. And guess what? Many patients who lose weight find that the pain goes away in their knees and backs, and they don't have the operation because they don't need it.

This is true as well with medications and the pain associated with these issues. Once the extra stress is lessened, the body feels better. Sleep apnea, hypertension, and diabetes are other examples of medical and surgical issues that often are improved or even resolved by simply taking care of you.

How is that for extra success? Think of saving all that time, rehabilitation, and discomfort simply by eating less. Just a thought!

The key here is reprogramming your thinking. You are in charge of your schedule and your time. Carve out time each day for a little bit of exercise, to prepare your own food in a healthier way, and to use the techniques I am teaching you in this book. You don't need to make this a big deal, just a real deal.

CHAPTER 30

Reprogramming Your Mind's Thermostat for Pain

The mind is intimately connected with your body and every nerve that carries impulses through it. These nerves are miraculous in that they allow you to feel, dance, see, type, experience the softness of a baby's cheek, and yes, be aware of pain and discomfort. They do this by sending impulses along their length, and remember, this impulse or stimulus is simply a message that there was a stimulation. Sometimes the stimulus may be a little stronger or a little less intense, but all the same, it is simply a stimulus wired to a specific part of your brain. Your little finger sends a stimulus to one part of the brain and your stomach, when it's hungry, to another. Want to know where your leg or wrist is in space, how it is positioned, or if there is a broken bone? Signals will be sent to the appropriate centers to let your brain know what's going on. The signals or impulses along the path of any nerve are all basically the same, but they go to different centers.

The centers that allow us to feel pain and discomfort are specific. They respond to a set of chemical messages that come from the nerves. The interesting thing about the pain center in the brain is that it has different levels of reactivity to the same signal depending on what else is going on. In other words, at different times, it takes more or less impulse to make the body and mind aware of its pain. Have you ever had a headache come and go, or something that you hurt such as a sprain or even a break? Sometimes it hurts a lot, and other times, even an hour later, it hurts a lot less. Some of this is whether you are focusing on it or not, and other times it has to do with the mind's interpretation of the stimulus that comes from the hurt area. That is correct; your mind judges the stimulus and determines its proper level of attention.

What we've found with meditation, mindful observation, and self-hypnosis is that we can actually reset the body's way of sensing things. Pain itself is our friend! Without pain we would not know to remove our hand from a hot stove or to take a splinter out of a sore foot before it blisters, becomes infected, and causes our bodies and bloodstream to become toxic. The pain is simply a warning sign in our body that something is wrong. Our stomach is full, and if we eat too much, it gets even more full in sensation or even painful from the dilation of the stomach lining and its neural sensory network. We need to stop eating or we feel like "we are going to burst." This is a sensation that most of us have ignored to our own dismay at one time or another.

As adults, or experienced big kids, we can train ourselves to be aware of these sensations. When you are very young and you don't understand where that discomfort is coming from in your belly, you might scream or cry. With potty training we come to understand that these impulses are not necessarily bad ones but rather signs to us that we better take care of business, at first in a diaper, and ultimately they serve us well when we learn to use the bathroom instead. Who said growing up was easy!

As an adult the next steps are understanding that sometimes you are full but in other circumstances, your stomach may be being assaulted by something internal, you may have eaten something too spicy or greasy, or perhaps you even have food poisoning.

When it comes to feeling and discomfort, we can reset this thermostat. This is not ignoring these warning sensations; it is learning how to interpret and use them without letting them overwhelm us. Remember, if pain is life-threatening, your subconscious mind will always protect you and not allow you to ignore it, but in most cases, resetting is easily and effectively achievable. When we use hypnosis for surgery, we are actually able to reset the mind's concept and expectation of how it will feel. You hear all kinds of stories from friends and professionals about what surgery is and what you will feel during and afterward. Remember this, every person is different. You will feel what your body experiences, and to a good extent, what you expect, and then decide how you will deal with that.

Yes, of course, it can make you sore or even very uncomfortable when someone does an operation on your body. It is in a sense an assault, a cut, but not that different from other experiences you have had in your life. But how you perceive that discomfort is very much an individual choice.

How do you see the surgery, as a healing process or as something that will brutalize or harm you? Your expectation and vision are very important—in fact how you experience it is really all that is important. If you have a fear of surgery, which is normal as an initial reaction, and feel it is going to harm you or make you miserable, you might want to rethink that surgery or find a way to address these concerns beforehand. If, on the other hand, you see it as a healing process and a way to make your life better and happier, then begin envisioning that. You don't need to be locked into thinking of surgery as a horrible process. It can actually be a very nice experience.

I find my patients often seem much more relaxed and comfortable than I am when they have an operation or procedure. In fact some days I am pretty sure I am more stressed than them. I believe this is because by the time my patients have surgery with me and they know our staff and have made a comfortable mutual decision to proceed, they turn over much of the worry to me and just go about their day.

Look at childbirth; some people love the experience and others feel it was an extreme challenge to deal with the pain. Personally having been with my wife at each of our children's deliveries, I am awed at the ability of women to take on this great gift as well as physical challenge. Some people afterward look back and wish they had been able to enjoy the whole experience a bit more with greater comfort. Why is this different for each person? They can go through the same amount of labor, the same number and intensity of contractions, the same dilation, the same size baby, and yet some people are comfortable, and others find the experience very uncomfortable. Others have babies in fields and in natural childbirth settings and feel wonderful. Some have told me that the overwhelming sense of joy and happiness at what they are producing overwhelms and overcomes that sense of pain. This is just one more thing we can learn from mothers;

love and joy are emotions that completely envelop the mind, and this is a wonderful way to distract the mind from the pain the body experiences. And even more fascinating is the fact that many women have more than one baby; it is worth it to them to redo the experience, and I have been told that the memory of pain generally fades while the sense of joy and fulfillment lasts a lifetime.

CHAPTER 31

Begin Your Preparation— The A, B, C...okay, and D

What to Expect in the Weeks before Surgery

A

First and foremost—share the fact that you are using medical meditation and self-hypnosis to help you have a more wonderful surgical experience with those close enough to you who really care, and only with those who believe in it. Don't ask opinions and don't ask for advice as to whether you should or should not do this; you've already made that decision—you're reading this book! But there are always people out there who will tell you that you cannot do something. Whether it is getting a job, passing a test, making enough money, getting that car, or whatever it is you're trying to do, there are those who will give you reasons not to if you tell people about it. Many people take great pleasure and comfort in telling you that you cannot do things, many times because they don't feel that they can. Others are well-meaning, trying to instill the wisdom they have gained in their lives from their own perspective...sometimes that of a person who thinks

"I can't" instead of "I can." In any case trust your instincts, trust the science that says most operations go without a hitch, and trust the fact that your body and mind are very powerful and can make a big difference in how your day goes.

B

Eliminate the naysayers immediately and completely. You may feel a little strange at the concept of trying to be in control of your mind and your life, but that's OK...no one has told you that you could until now. I am telling you; you can remain in control and give yourself a much more wonderful experience.

Hear all the positive and avoid the naysayers! Don't listen to the negatives and negative people. This includes medical professionals!

Yes, informed consent is necessary, legally for the docs and to an extent for you as a patient to know what can go wrong with surgery, medication, and other treatments. Of course in your initial research you should learn the up-and-down sides of any treatment.

But once you have researched the surgery and/or treatment and made an intelligent and informed decision to have surgery or use the medications, let go of the worry and concern about the side effects, complications, and/or diatribes you will get from nurses, docs, anesthesiologists, and other treating professionals. If possible have an advocate who can read these releases you need to sign and complication lists—that happen in reality to few—and don't rehash the lists of possible problems; you did that at the beginning, and that is why you decided to go ahead...now let it go.

This way you can focus on the positives, feeling great, and healing.

I have family members who've undergone some very serious treatments. I took on the advocate role and heard all these possible issues for them. This allowed them to focus on the healing, and by and large they never experienced the possible side effects of the procedures, treatments, or medications because there was no expectation. I still could watch for problems and validate things if they felt them but also helped them believe that healing was easy, and though, as with everyone, being sick or having surgery can be tiring and stressful or make you a little sore, if you do not expect it to interfere with your life; it likely will not!

This world is filled with mixed messages and distorted facts concerning surgery, medications, self-healing, and many treatments, some valid and some distorted beyond comprehension. All of it doesn't matter. You are now in charge.

You'll find over the next few weeks as you begin practicing these exercises that you will become better and better at bringing yourself into this relaxed state. By the time you reach the operating room or start your medication or treatment regime, you'll have brought yourself into this relaxed state many times and know that it is as simple as slowing down your breathing.

The same holds true for controlling your own pain or lessening medications. As you practice and understand how great it feels to be in control of your own mind and body, you'll notice that you feel better, you are less dependent on a pill, and you are able to duplicate the effects of those meds and need them less.

C

Know that you will feel great and have a wonderful day. The first thing you will find when you begin practicing these techniques is that you feel better. If nothing else, you're giving yourself twenty minutes a day to rest and relax and let go. You're reminding your subconscious mind that you want to be happy, healthy, and feel great. The fact is, you actually began your healing process already when you took the first step with your decision to read this book.

Here's what you might expect to feel:

- **-You'll begin to feel that you are in control of your world—inner and outer.** You will begin to feel and understand that you can make yourself happy, healthy, and relaxed, and you will begin to feel happier, healthier, and more relaxed.

- **-You'll feel less pressure concerning making yourself feel comfortable and relaxed.** You may notice things like your blood pressure going down, you may begin to see some aches and pains abate, and you may find you have more energy because this is giving you extra rest and your body extra time to recuperate from the daily traumas it faces.

- **-You begin to see and understand that you can relax and let go.** You can bring yourself to a state where you are better able to let go of many of the small, minor worries and concerns in your life and also take control over many others.

• **-You begin to understand that taking time to take care of you does not lose you time but gains you time.** You become more efficient and happier, and you will feel better throughout your day. You find that you have more time and more energy to get more done because you've taken time to relax and take care of you. You also begin to understand that everyone has this ability. You and every other individual who can think and dream can utilize these techniques, and there are no limits to what you can achieve. More than that you will realize very quickly how easy this is to do. Everyone and anyone can do it. I've induced trances thousands of times in patients, and I can tell you it is predictable, easy, and it really works. You begin to see the extra bounce of happiness and energy as you simply live your life.

D

Don't worry about if it's working or not or how well it's working. People have successfully used relaxation techniques, meditation, hypnosis, and prayer for thousands of years. It is all the same. You'll have some days where you feel absolutely wonderful and others where you feel nothing is happening. It doesn't matter; just keep doing what you are doing. You'll begin to see gradual and progressive changes in you and your life as well as the way you feel. Don't worry about if you're more relaxed or less relaxed, you are simply learning to handle stress and challenges by focusing on the moment, not the day-to-day events of life. The key is you'll begin to gain more control, not of the world and life necessarily but most importantly over yourself and how you react to what goes on outside of you.

Let go of the how, why, when, and where; just let it happen. Don't worry, it's working!

It is certainly normal, and every one of us has doubts and concerns and wonders how good we are at this and how well it works. I've been doing this for over thirty years and work with professional societies that train individuals to do hypnosis; I have trained the trainers. I know that every one of us has questions. It is human nature. Just let go and notice how much better you feel, how your life begins to change, and how you begin to understand that you actually have control over what is happening around you and to your body—control over how you react to stresses to your body, minor traumas and minor aches, and yes, even surgery when it happens. Even if you decide not to use this at all for your surgery or to use the medications exactly as recommended or just go with stronger anesthesia and don't use this, you will already have programmed your mind, and it will make a difference. So... let go, or as Bobby McFerrin says, "Don't Worry, Be Happy"!

You will have days where you feel nothing is going right, and you will break one or all my special rules for relaxation, medication control and surgery—that's perfectly OK!

Understand this is a process, like life. You will have days when you feel out of control and stressed, you will stub your toe, and it will hurt, and you can't make it go away. Someone will hurt your feelings, scare you or make you doubt yourself and you will be stressed out—that's OK. None of us is meant to be perfect. We are in this world to experience being human, spiritual beings in a physical body. We are here to experience discomfort, happiness, suffering, love, anger, and everything in between. If you didn't, you wouldn't be human.

When you do get frustrated, though, you always have a choice. You can either berate yourself, be upset, give up, and tell yourself that you will never be able to relax and master this...

Or:

You can just simply go back to the beginning. Every time you do this, it is the first time, and each time is different. So let yourself go, count yourself in, and relax once again. Remind yourself that every day, every minute, and every hour is a new start. You get to do it again and again, and when you screw up or don't do it just the way you wanted to, keep going. Trust me, it works.

Barry Sears, the author of *The Zone Diet*, based the diet on eating approximately every five hours. He gives some specifics on the best way to eat, but he makes a very good point. He says that even if you screw up, eat everything in the world that you shouldn't, go completely off the diet—five hours later you get to start again! It's the same thing with medical meditation and self-hypnosis. But instead of five hours later, you get to do it five minutes or five seconds later. You can always bring yourself back in control of your inner world simply by sitting back, closing your eyes, slowing your breathing, and relaxing. You may find your improvements are in small increments or great leaps. It doesn't matter as long as each day you strive to be a little better than the day before; that's all any of us can do.

CHAPTER 32

The Four Golden Rules

Rule Number 1

When you feel stressed, "put yourself in"—simply use the techniques you've learned here to take care of you whenever you feel a need (put yourself in medical meditation). Simply breathe, close your eyes, and let yourself drift into your own medical meditation and self-hypnosis!

Rule Number 2

"Put yourself in" whenever you want, not just when and because you think you should.

Rule Number 3

Take time for your medical meditation, relaxation, and self-hypnosis happily, guilt-free, and completely—enjoy the time you have given yourself.

Rule Number 4

Don't miss a day! It is really that simple!

Can this really be that easy?

Remember this: The mind can only focus on one thing at a time. If you see yourself as happy, healthy, and relaxed, enjoying the day, focused intently on something that you enjoy or find pleasurable or my voice, then that is all you will see, hear, sense, and feel. The surgery will go on, and you will know nothing of it. Pain medication doses will be skipped, and you will suddenly realize you need less. Your subconscious mind will handle keeping your blood pressure stable and your heart rate steady. The correct hormones for healing and comfort are secreted as your body protects and cares for itself while you are doing exactly what you should be for healing and decreasing discomfort. You begin to heal even while the operation is going on; that is what your subconscious does. You, in the meantime, can just enjoy the day as a very nice, comfortable experience. Remember, with medical meditation it is of no consequence what goes on around you; all your mind knows is to take care of you, with or without your input. It's not much different than having a massage. Initially you may be aware someone is massaging your body, but many times, you'll just fall asleep (usually into alpha relaxation, meditation mistaken for sleep). The kneading and active pushing and prodding on those sore points and muscles will go on, but you pretty much sleep through it. No different with surgery or opioid medication!

CHAPTER 33

Let's Go Over Your Plan

1.
You will practice daily so that you are ready for the big day.

2.
By the time you reach the hospital and the operating suite, you will be in your own wonderful world of self-hypnosis, enjoying and relaxing while everything goes on around you.

3.
During the procedure you will be simply letting go, listening to the audio, and letting your body do what it does best: taking care of you.

4.
When the operation is over, you will be awakening, feeling refreshed and happy, already on your way to healing. Your medical

self-hypnosis will continue to work with you throughout the healing process.

No matter whether you augment this with a local anesthetic,
a sedation anesthesia, or even a general anesthesia, it does not
matter. The experience will overall be more pleasant, you will
recover more quickly and easily, and you will enjoy it with a better outcome, knowing before it even starts that your healing is
going to occur.

Remember: The same holds true for medication and therapy
treatments! Once your mind's expectation is that you will feel
better the need for medication will become less and less.

Frequently Asked Questions

What if the medical meditation and self-hypnosis don't work?

Nothing lost and much gained. At least you were relaxed when
you went in. The hospital and doctors have many medications
and other ways to make you comfortable. They will need less of
them when you use the medical meditation, and perhaps none
at all. But they are always there as a backup. If nothing else, you
and your body are better prepared for the operation. You have
made a plan, and every plan has options for success. You win
either way because you and your mind and body are prepared
for a great day, and you have begun your healing before you even
arrive at the hospital!

The same holds true for medications. If you have decided to
lessen or even stop medications (with your doc's blessing that it is

safe to do so), you may well run into challenges or setbacks. This is fine since the goal is to enhance the effectiveness of medical treatments and eventually allow your body to duplicate their effects. Either way you make the process of feeling better and healing easier and more pleasurable. That is correct; there is a feeling of empowerment and enhancement of your life when you take charge of your healing and the events in your life.

What if there is a problem and I need to wake up?

You will always awaken if necessary. Although your conscious mind is asleep, your subconscious mind is wide awake. If you need to awaken, you will arouse and do whatever it is you need to do to help you or the doctors. Once you have completed that, you will simply go back into your relaxed state.

Remember, self-hypnosis is exactly that; you are in control and in charge. Although it feels very much like sleep, your subconscious always is aware and takes care of you. It is aware of your surroundings and will respond as necessary to whatever is needed.

What if everyone else in the hospital doesn't believe in what I'm doing?

My best advice is to find a surgeon and team that allow you to do what you are doing—or just do it anyway; it is not their concern and will make no difference to them except perhaps in seeing afterward how easily you tolerated whatever the procedure as compared to others. Whether they believe it or not will have no influence on how you do. As long as they respect your wishes and allow you to listen to the audio (ideally but not necessarily if the situation dictates you cannot) through the procedure, this will not affect you one way or the other. The one caveat here is that it would be nice to be able to request of them that they give you positive suggestions when you awaken, such as "All went well" or "How are you feeling?" or "How was your nap?" Ask them to avoid negative suggestions like "Are you having any pain?"

"How do you feel" is just as good, and if you do have discomfort, you will still tell them, and they will give you something for it! The key is to maintain a positive attitude, and if you do so, no matter what goes on around you, all will be well.

CHAPTER 34

Let's Begin the Actual Program of Setting Your Mind up for a Wonderfully Happy Day

The Dalai Lama in his book *The Art of Happiness* talks about compassion. Compassion is important—for others, and equally important, if not more so, for yourself. No one, absolutely no one, knows better how to take care of you than you. You must be compassionate for any suffering that you go through as well as the suffering of others.

Understanding and having compassion for your doctor, the nurses, and the staff of the operating room will help too. Being nice to them and realizing that their job is stressful is essential. This doesn't mean you need to go out of your way and bring them flowers or donuts, but it does mean that understanding they have stress may help you in dealing with some of the ways they act or the things they may say or do. The same holds true for your personal doctor or medical professional; they are people, and remember that their goal is to help you heal. Don't take things in a personal way, just be and let them be and do their job, as long as they are not hurting you or sincerely upsetting you. If so there are ways to let them know, and one of them is simply to say, "I'm afraid," or "I need to understand," or "I need your help to relax and get through this day." Most of the time these people do not realize how they are coming across, or frankly, they are simply overwhelmed and sometimes so stressed about getting their own stuff done that they're not even aware of you or your feelings. Although you are the patient, very often a little smile and a little openness goes a long way. Being compassionate for yourself is all about understanding that yes, this is an experience, like many others you have in your life, but one which is anxiety-provoking. Anyone who can help you be less anxious and more relaxed will be your friend and ally, and a great benefit to you in getting through the day.

A funny story about compassion:

My father, as mentioned before, was a clinical psychologist, and during his final year of life his heart and other systems in his body finally began to fail. But his basic love of people and passion for helping them never wavered. It was always amusing to hear the stories he brought home about the hospital staff who took care of him. His room often became a therapy office for staff to the extent that many of the nurses and doctors greeted us when we came to visit him, thanking us for sharing him with them. He literally did therapy with many, and nights were not generally restful for him, since he was usually up talking to them through the night. He used to joke that a hospital is no place to get some rest!

One day as we approached his room, we heard exquisite and resonating flamenco dancing taps all the way down the hall. We had no idea why this would be happening in the hospital and were astounded to see a famous flamenco dancer practicing in the hallway. It seems he'd had a heart attack and was quite depressed at the thought that the return to dance would be too strenuous on his heart. Well, of course he had met Dad, and they talked a lot about heart disease, and comparatively speaking, this fine gentleman realized his situation was not as bad as Dad's, so he might be OK. That realization came out of his "therapy session" and a little hypnotic suggestion from Dad. So he decided to test it out, and soon afterward he was discharged and returned to performing.

I tell this story not to talk about Dad, which our family loves to do, but more so as an example of how we affect those around us every day, and the truth was, the staff loved Dad, and he got superb care till the day he decided it was time for him to go. He also dealt with his pain more easily and nobly. The reason: He treated people kindly and empathized with their pain instead of focusing on his own.

CHAPTER 35

Your Program

The audios and the techniques in this book are medically based and proven to work in real clinical situations with real people. They work, whether you are facing an opioid or medication dependence, stress, pain, a medical procedure, or a major surgery. These techniques and exercises prepare you for a daily life of single events or a one-time life event. The methods and effectiveness are the same, and all are based on consistency in learning a technique that allows you to be better in charge of your body and how you feel no matter what is going on outside yourself.

There is an old story about a musician who travels to New York City to find the famed Carnegie Hall. He's never been to New York before and wants to become a famous violinist. His vision is to play there, and he wants to see this glorious place and burn the image in his mind. He's wandering around the city and trying to find his way, completely without direction or a plan, with his beloved violin tucked under his arm. A taxi is stopped near him, and he figures, what better advice can I get than from a taxi driver? They always know where everything is and how to get there. He knocks on the window gently, and the cabbie looks over. He rolls down the window and the musician asks, "How do I get to Carnegie Hall?"

The cabbie sizes him up and pauses a moment, then replies, "Practice, man, practice." Sounds easy and it really is that simple— put your mind to it, and it manifests!

OK. You know how to do it, you know what it's about, but how do you make it happen? One word—practice!

Remember to have a wonderful day taking care of you or in the operating room, with a new way to take care of you and/or gain back control over your healing and medication needs. All you do is continue to own your program:

1. Prepare, prepare, prepare—you've already started—simply continue your program.

2. Do it your way. You've chosen what feels right to you; stay with it.

3. Remember...you are the boss of you. You will heal because you choose to.

4. Trust your inner knowing.

Remember, medical meditation and self-hypnosis are simply fixed, focused states of attention.

What do you want to focus on while you are having your procedure? If it were me, it would be on that beach or in the woods in a quiet place or on some mountaintop. The last place I'd want to think about being is where I am. That's what this is about. When you direct your attention in a manner that brings you someplace else, you are, for all practical intents and purposes, there and not here.

Remember that your mind can only focus on one thing at a time, so if it's focused on feeling great, relaxed, and happy, then everything else that's going on around you just doesn't really exist, at least not to your mind and body. Just like children, we as adults can be distracted through our imaginations, and the more distracted you are and the more vivid that daydream, the better you feel; you literally create a reality for your subconscious and your inner world that brings you only smiles and peace. Your focus on happiness allows no place for any of the unpleasantries that may exist. Reality is only in your mind.

CHAPTER 36

A Little Exercise for Your Mind: The Perfect Day

Here is an exercise I would like you to begin doing to prepare for your day in the hospital or for any medical procedure you may be getting ready for.

Take a few moments to sit down and turn off any distractions, your phone, computer and begin to slow your breathing as you already know how. Allow your eyelids to gently close and allow yourself to drift into your personal relaxed state. You can use any of the techniques in the audios or choose simply to breathe and let go.

Allow your neck, shoulders and face to relax and feel any tensions or stresses drain out with each out breath. Do this for a few minutes and then imagine your perfect day. Perhaps you are in your favorite place, laying on a beach, in a park or simply relaxing anywhere you like. See yourself completely at ease and just enjoying having no responsibility or interruptions, just being and breathing letting your mind and body relax and enjoy.

Once you are there, take a few more minutes and simply breathe and enjoy the experience... and when you are ready, simply count yourself back awake from one until 10 reminding yourself that you are happy, healthy and relaxed, feeling great. When you reach 10, open your eyes and enjoy the peace you have created.

Use this image of your perfect day any time and perhaps revisit that place during your meditations and in the following session.

If you do these exercises on a regular daily basis, you will become better and better at them. If you don't have a lot of time before the big day, then simply do them as many times as you can, but the key is repetition, which creates subconscious learning. You've studied for tests, shot a basketball or practiced dancing, learned to write—in fact everything you have learned in your life required you to practice. This is no different. Listening to me on the audio will allow you exactly what you desire.

It does not matter if it makes it 5 percent or 50 percent better; it is still a great asset for you and your healing, not to mention your medical team. Then you can lie back and let your doctor do the rest!

Remember what I said about practice—your mind certainly will.

When we go over things and practice them, we become better and better at achieving our goal. When we repeat ideas and beliefs in our subconscious mind, it accepts them more and more as reality.

Using these techniques for surgery, sleep or control of your discomfort - you control your response to stress and also the secretion of those hormones in your brain, (the endorphins and enkephalins, the "feel-good hormones") that allow you to feel better, sleep better by producing your own melatonin…and yes, decrease pain by secreting your body's own internally produced morphine, the most powerful painkiller known to mankind. All by simply relaxing and letting your body do what it knows naturally how to do…to take care of you!

You will, without any active input or effort, automatically bring yourself to a state where everything will indeed be all right, and you will awaken from your operation happy, healthy, and relaxed. The more you use the audio portion of this book and practice, the easier it will be for your mind to bring you to that place and allow this to happen without a second thought. This applies to the day of surgery or to any day; whether you choose to use it to decrease the need for medications or deal with one specific challenging day, it is all the same. You are in complete control of your mind and body simply by relaxing.

Here is your OR session. This session can be used for healing and for your day in surgery. It has the option for you to play on repeat and this will take you back to the beginning so you can stay in as long as you desire. Once you are in the recovery room and ready to come back awake, you will simply count yourself up from one until 10 and you will be awake, alert and relaxed.

This session can also be used for dealing with pain, anxiety, sleep radiation, chemotherapy or to program your mind for healing with less medication.

Listen to the Audio!
Audio #4:
Medical Meditation for Surgery and Healing
***A Relaxing, Repeating Session for Surgery ,Comfort and Healing

CHAPTER 37

Belief and Programming Yourself

Question: What if I'm having trouble visualizing and seeing this? What if I'm afraid I can't do it?

That is normal. All of us worry that "it may not work for me." The fact is, whether you feel you are doing something or not does not matter because simply taking time to let go and breathing slowly are all your subconscious mind needs to prompt it to take care of you. Over the years I have had hundreds of people say to me, "I didn't feel anything," or "I never went into meditation" while they were in my group, and I had hypnotized them.

They would say, "I never was out," even though they were sometimes snoring or sound asleep; it is a common misconception. They were always amazed though when they looked at their watch and could not figure out where the past hour had gone. That is correct: When I asked them how long they thought they had tried to relax, they would guess five or ten minutes when in reality they had completely relaxed for an hour.

Remember, everyone visualizes, and everyone daydreams. It's no different than drifting off to sleep at night except that you decide when you want to go there. That state just before you drift off to sleep is meditation. So essentially you have been doing this every night of your life; it's simply doing the same thing at a different time. Meditation and self-hypnosis are simply daydreaming except you purposefully bring yourself there. After you've practiced these techniques a few times, listening to my voice guide you through it, you will basically know how to bring yourself into this state. Of course you can continue to use the audios; there is nothing wrong with that and many people prefer guided meditation. But the fact is, each time you do it again and/or listen to me and my voice guide you through it, you will become better and better. No matter what, you gain all the benefits no matter how deep you do or do not go. Together we will walk and talk you through this, and soon you will be self-empowered, stronger, more confident, and more capable of taking care of you.

Question: Sometimes I feel like I'm not hearing you and I'm sleeping, but when you count me up to awaken, I always wake up. Is this OK?

Remember, deep meditation and hypnosis are sleep states for your conscious mind and awake states for your subconscious mind. While your conscious mind, that take-care-of-details busy mind, goes to sleep and rests and lets go of some of its daily worries and stresses, your subconscious mind remains wide awake and takes in everything it hears. The subconscious mind has one single purpose: to take care of you. If you fall asleep while listening to the audio and me, that's OK. No harm is done.

The above said, ideally I would not use this to go to sleep all the time because you will gain only partial benefit. The ideal is to practice this in a position where you will not go completely to sleep. A good time to do this is during the day, midday, or even in the early evening or first thing in the morning. As long as you are practicing sometime during the day, if you want to sleep and use this to sleep as well, that's perfectly okay, but also do it during the day when you will be awake enough for the subconscious mind to allow your suggestions and desires to be reinforced. This is not just a relaxation technique; it is a tool to use to help your subconscious mind understand clearly what you want and how you want to feel. Remember, this is your chance to place your deepest desires in your subconscious so that your subconscious can make them reality.

So bottom line...don't sweat it if you fall asleep; your body needed to rest. You still will get great benefit. And each day, each hour, is a new beginning!

CHAPTER 38

Dealing with Doubt, Stress, and Worry

I do feel like I'm beginning to relax, but when I'm faced with a real situation like surgery or lessening my medications, will this work?

Yes, it will! Again, practice is key, but also remember that if you do get a little anxious, you are not doing this all alone. We all worry, doubt, and stress over the decisions we make. Perhaps even at this point you are wondering if you made the right decision to have surgery or use the medications or drugs you are taking or plan to. Your mind continues to question decisions and go through the positive and negative scenarios. This is a good thing because thinking any choice through is a great way to be sure a decision is right for you. But once you make a decision, based on all the information above we have discussed in this book…let it go. You've done your homework; now it is time to relax and prepare yourself to get the greatest benefit from your choice that you can.

You are certainly able to, and indeed if you have any concern, probably should augment these techniques with a little medication. It may be a general anesthetic, a sedation anesthesia, or a novocaine block to help numb up the area even more than with your mind. The same holds true for medication use; you can prolong the time between medication doses, decrease the amount you take (i.e., cut the pill in half) or see how you do without it as long as your doc says it is safe.

So just think, if you are doing this well already just by doing the audio and relaxing a bit, how great it will be when you get a little extra push from a medicine, which allows you to go deeper into your subconscious state. The combination of using modern technology along with your own brain is an extraordinary thing, and you will be surprised at how wonderfully the two work together.

CHAPTER 39

A Grounding Technique

There are many ways to bring yourself into your relaxed state. Some people like to stare at a fixed point, others at the back of their eyelids. You may find rubbing two fingers together or rubbing the top of your head works. Some play with their hair; this doesn't work for me since I cut mine off, but I do enjoy rubbing the top of my bald head, which is relaxing to me. You may choose just to touch a finger to the side of your nose or make yourself yawn by opening your mouth wide. For some it is as simple as remembering to take a deep breath and let it out slowly.

The key is, come up with what your little trigger is, and begin playing with that and using it. Whenever you want to bring yourself to your relaxed state, do that either by touching two fingers together, touching your arm or the side of your nose with your finger, or making a fist and relaxing it or any of the other ideas I've given you above. If you begin to feel any anxiety or stress or that things are not completely in control, go back to your little trigger and use it.

In hypnosis we call this reinforcing or anchoring a thought. Simply bring yourself to your relaxed state and tell your subconscious mind you wish to associate this behavior with re-laxing and say "whenever I do this, I will immediately take a deep breath and let go." Then simply perform the simple trigger you have chosen. This way not only do you visualize that sense of healing, but you can also use a physical element to reinforce and bond that emotion to a physical action. You can then use that, if you like, at a time you feel anxious or stressed.

A card for your doctor:

Here is a card for you to give to your anesthesiologist, nurses, and doctor.

> *Hello, I am having surgery today, and I use medical meditation and relaxation to help with making this a calm and happy day—for me and for you as well.*
>
> *Could you please help by doing the following:*
>
> - *Allow me to relax and rest as long as it is safe and not inconvenient for you or your team.*
>
> - *Please do not mention the word "pain," but ask me simply, "How do you feel?" or "How are you doing?" instead. This helps me to focus on feeling great and to enhance the effectiveness of your medications.*

- *Please allow me to listen to my audio relaxation with my headphones before and if at all possible, during the procedure... and after. If you need to interrupt me to ask me something or for my safety, of course this is absolutely OK.*

- *Although I may appear asleep, I will be awake and aware enough to answer questions and do what you need me to do, and though I look like I am sleeping, I am really using medical meditation to relax.*

- *Lastly, you and your team are very special. Thank you for indulging me and allowing me to help you to take care of me.*

CHAPTER 40

Self-Anesthesia
Taking Care of You
Because You Can

I had a patient once who was a longshoreman. He was a very nice chap and came from a breed of very tough, hard-working guys. He didn't have a lot of money and came to me one day telling me that he had a significant problem with his arm. We talked about what he needed to have done, and he told me he really didn't have a problem with handling discomfort. I told him that was great and that there were a number of ways to decrease discomfort and tolerate procedures from an orthopedic point of view. We talked about self-hypnosis and relaxation. Then he told me he had his own way of taking care of himself.

It seems he had gone to a dentist, and the dentist told him that all his teeth needed to come out because of a significant gum disease. The dentist quoted him thousands of dollars to go in and pull all his teeth from the top of his mouth. He wasn't very happy about this, and further he really didn't have the money. He told me he went to the hardware store and bought himself a nice pair of pliers. He then bought a bottle of good rum. He drank until he was at a very relaxed state and then visualized in his mind saving all that money and proceeded to pull out all his teeth with the pliers. It's not the way I'd recommend doing things, but suffice to say if you put your mind to something you can make it happen. He said he tolerated the procedure very well. He had no help, no problems, and saved himself a trip to the dentist.

Every one of us isn't a longshoreman, and certainly I don't recommend self-care in the way my patient did. On the other hand, he taught me something: No matter where you are in life and what the situation, you can always maintain control.

The main reason we use anesthesia in the operating room is to relax patients so that it is easier to do the job we do. Yes, there is a component of the anesthesia that relieves discomfort, and this can often be handled simply with the addition of a local anesthetic. But anesthesia itself basically puts you to sleep or relaxes you to a point where your body doesn't really feel or care, and basically isn't aware of what's going on. It can be achieved in many ways and for different operations, different levels and depths of anesthesia and relaxation are required. What it really does is quiet your conscious mind, the part that is aware of the day-to-day and minute-to-minute happenings of your life.

There are many operations and procedures that simply require you to relax a bit, and there is often literally no discomfort, or any sense of discomfort is eliminated by the use of an injection of novacaine or another similar local anesthetic. Dental surgery is a great example. If you relax you can undergo a surgery or procedure and literally have no discomfort at all, just as I experienced with my dentist. Remember, hypnosis is not a sleep state but rather one where your subconscious mind is in a state of heightened awareness. My conscious mind was asleep, but my subconscious knew what was going on. I was able to keep my mouth open and not worry about gagging and experienced a rewarding fascination with the operation and how it went. I found myself drifting in and out of an awareness that this was going on but had no discomfort whatsoever. I never took a pill, needed any medication, or had a bit of discomfort throughout the procedure nor afterward.

In fact dental anesthesia is mainly about reducing anxiety, so of course, medical meditation and self-hypnosis has been highly effective—not just in anxiety reduction, but for those who choose to do so, it is fairly easy to instill a sense of numbness or tingling in the area of the jaw simply by brushing the facial nerve ten times and allowing an altered sensation to impart. It is very useful, even if you still use the local anesthetic, since you likely will not even feel the local being injected.

Listen once again to the Healing Session – Healing Sand.

CHAPTER 41

Lets Talk Anesthesia

There are many types of anesthesia and ways to be relaxed. There is sedation anesthesia, which relaxes you using medications such as Propofol, Valium, or Versed. This allows you to be in a sleepy state, relaxing your muscles and your mind, allowing your body to completely relax. You can reproduce the effect of these medications using medical meditation or self-hypnosis, and even better and more important, you can enhance their effectiveness if you choose to use them, even on a limited basis. I find with my patients who choose to use light sedation or conscious, twilight-type anesthesia as it's sometimes called, that they're in that relaxed state even before any medications are given since they began their medical meditation and relaxation upon arrival to the hospital. In fact when they get to the operating room, medical students (and frankly, sometimes the anesthesia staff) often ask if they have given my patient medication already. The nurses who have worked with me before tell them, "No, that's just Scott's way." They know that my patients generally need less sedation to achieve the same effectiveness, which is safer, and the nicest part is they have fewer complications and fewer side effects from the medicine, and when they are ready to wake up, there is really not as much medication to come out of their system. They recover much more easily and are able to go home more quickly and awaken much more comfortably, without the nausea or other side effects that occur sometimes with these medications. It is safer because they are breathing more on their own and it is easier for everyone involved. In fact it's also cheaper because less anesthesia medication needs to be given. But they are equally if not more comfortable than the patients who do not use these techniques. It is a true win-win!

Local with Sedation and Twilight Anesthesia

This is injecting a numbing substance such as Marcaine or Lidocaine into an area after giving the patient something to relax them. In my patients I do this after they are already relaxed, so many times they never even feel the injection at all. I like using local anesthetic along with sedation with medical meditation and self-hypnosis. Generally for the more complex cases, we have an anesthesiologist in the room to deliver these medications. In cases like this the anesthesiologist or anesthetist gives the patient something to sedate them, or make them sleepy, augmenting the medical meditation. We then add the local anesthetic via injecting the area to be operated or in some cases a nerve block is done to numb an entire extremity.

We do many procedures in the office and often with just medical meditation along with a light muscle relaxer and the local anesthetic. I use it all the time! Patients in most cases are so relaxed that they know no difference between an alcohol swab on the skin and the actual insertion of the needle. By the time they are ready to have the injection and the anesthesia infiltrated, they are very relaxed and have essentially numbed the area themselves. You already know that this is possible and something you will and can do, even without thinking about it or knowing you are doing it.

General Anesthesia

This is completely going to sleep when the anesthesiologist brings you to a deep relaxed state. Again remember, patients feel and hear under anesthesia. The anesthesia is simply imparting a deep sleep state. When your body is relaxed enough, it is not aware of what is going on, so it really doesn't feel much—that is, the body has no conscious awareness of any discomfort or what is going on. But to be sure, patients under anesthesia do feel. This is why other medications are used along with the sleep anesthetic to help decrease the body's reaction to major procedures. While you sleep your subconscious mind still takes care of you, and that is the part of your mind that reacts.

When you use medical meditation and self-hypnosis, your expectation is to feel good so once you are asleep the hypnotic suggestions continue, and you really feel quite comfortable. Not only are you feeling comfortable while you relax but your subconscious mind is already healing you, sending the correct messages through your hormones to your body for optimal healing. Your psyche is also constantly reminded as well that you are going to feel good, your healing is occurring already, and that you will awaken feeling wonderful, relaxed, and refreshed. What a great way to start your day after the operation is done and a success!

It has been shown by clinical studies that under hypnosis specifically, the immune system is enhanced in its effectiveness, so you are already fighting any infections, if they might be brewing, even before they start. Further, your body relaxes, your blood pressure stays low and your muscles remain relaxed - making the operation easier, as well as decreasing the need for more anesthesia.

Here's the bottom line:

You have the choice! You can use medical meditation and self-hypnosis, sedation, general anesthesia, or all of the above. You are in control. The key is not that you need to avoid the use of modern medicine. Modern medicine and its chemicals are wonderful. But you can use less, have fewer side effects and complications, and feel better than most who go through surgery because you are in control, and you get the benefits without the side effects of whatever type anesthesia you choose. Between minimal dosing and mind preparation, you win all around. That's the beauty of what you're doing.

CHAPTER 42

Questions about Anesthesia

Can I have surgery without any anesthesia?

Yes, you can. My father in fact did hypnosis for the first cesarean section in New York state, utilizing hypnosis in a woman who could not tolerate anesthesia. No other anesthetic. This feat has been repeated many times. A cesarean section is surgery, and yet no pain or discomfort was noted. It's not for everyone, but it certainly works and when indicated is a wonderful alternative. Even more powerful is the use of medical meditation with limited anesthesia or other techniques such as epidurals. Everything you now know applies; it is safer, equally effective, kinder, and in the case of childbirth, allows the whole experience to be more enjoyable and comfortable for the mom, the baby, and the medical professionals helping deliver the baby.

And you now know that the same is true for surgeries, especially procedures that do not require a very deep muscle dissection—these are ideal for this. Even major surgeries can be done utilizing only hypnosis, but don't try this without the guidance of

175

a medical professional who is very familiar with the options and who also is prepared to help you implement plan B if you need a little extra help.

On the other hand, why should you only use medical meditation or self-hypnosis for a major procedure? My preference for my patients is they have an anesthesiologist in the operating room for any major procedure. They can utilize just the right amount, which is usually less, anesthesia, and the rest is handled by the patient's subconscious using their medical meditation/hypnosis. Your anesthesiologist can judge how much anesthesia you will need and can gauge this. The bottom line is this—use what you've learned to make the day great, and have a professional oversee any additional medication or anesthetic as you request it, or it is needed. The result is predictable, since you're using less than others need, therefore you have fewer complications and side effects.

The same holds true for those of you who are working on limiting your use of medications or modifying the meds you may need for relief from pain, stress, or sleep. Adding your body and mind's own resources to good medical treatment allows you to be in control and limit your need for medications and subsequently limit your suffering from side effects, oversedation, or dependency. You regain control of you and your life, and let the opioids find their natural place as a rarely necessary addition.

How long will it take for me to get good enough to use this?

I find that between the sixth and eighth session of practicing these techniques on a regular basis, patients are ready to really utilize these techniques. That said, I have used them with patients who listen to my audios for the first time the day of their surgery and others who have minimal exposure to them. Most of them find these a great help, and to my recollection, in the past twenty years I cannot think of any who did not find some benefit. I am still surprised at how many people with literally no experience slip so easily into a deep, hypnotic, relaxed state and gain extraordinary relief and peace during and after their procedures.

Obviously the more you do this, the better prepared your subconscious mind is to utilize these techniques. But you don't have to be a "expert at hypnosis." Also, remember everyone can do this. It is simply daydreaming, letting go and believing, knowing that you have the same ability as every other person. If you can imagine, if you can visualize in any way, and everyone can, everyone who's ever daydreamed—you can do this. Practice is key, and the more you practice the stronger your belief, and that's what the exercises in this book are for. Leave the rest to me. As Milton Erickson, the famous psychologist and hypnotist, said, "My voice will go with you wherever you go." We will do this together to help you heal and have a wonderful experience.

Distractions—How to Keep It Going in the Hospital!

OK, you've made it to the big day. You're there and everything is going right. You've carefully planned and gotten yourself a nice relaxing morning, not rushing, and are at the hospital well on time. You may even have begun listening to the preparatory audio on the way while someone else drove and you just relaxed. But as you get to the hospital, if that completely normal sense of slight anxiety creeps into your head...here's what you do.

Remember that all our doubts, worries, and fears are reflex thoughts that we've learned. They have been created by those who are professional worriers or sensationalism generators. They are not real. As a child you were invincible; everything you thought and daydreamed was reality. Your dragons, Prince or Princess Charming, protector, and superheroes were all as real as the nose on your face. This is still in you and still reality. You are your own superhero and knight in shining armor, and as long as you continue to know that you are in control of your mind and body, everything will go your way. You've already given your doc and medical team permission to take care of the rest; you just have to take care of your thoughts. *Remember that these techniques are not just for a surgery day. They are for however long afterward you want to use them and for whatever stresses or discomforts come up. They help with healing and with overall health. They are also excellent for dealing with long-term pain issues, sleep problems, and the stresses and anxieties of daily life. Basically when you think about it, why not relax any time you have a chance? Life gets better, and you become happier and healthier and can enjoy each hour and every day more!*

Go back and repeat the Quick In-Out Session.

Triggers

We spoke about triggers a little earlier. Perhaps you would like a little reminder, a trigger for bringing back your relaxed state anytime and anywhere...

After using the techniques I've taught you, once you're relaxed, you may want to add a suggestion to your subconscious mind that it will relax whenever you do a certain action. You may choose what your trigger might be if you want to create one for your special day, or frankly, for every day and any time you choose to let go a little.

So choose something that resonates with you. It could be as simple as an extra deep "in" breath or perhaps a light touch in a certain area—rubbing two fingers together, touching your nose, or perhaps gently rubbing the top of your head (this one used to drive my wife crazy when I would do it, but now she rubs my head if she sees I am stressed) or maybe playing with your hair; whatever it is you decide could be your little secret trigger, do it. Now see yourself relaxing as you do this, and see it relaxing you even further. Tell yourself that whenever you wish to relax and bring yourself to this wonderful, safe, and peaceful state, this physical act will allow you to relax and let go. Practice imprinting this and see yourself happy, healthy, and relaxed whenever you do it. You'll likely find that by using this little trick, you will be able to decrease anxiety and stress whenever and wherever you choose.

Yay! You're in the recovery room. It's all done, and you did great.

CHAPTER 43

Let's Talk about the Recovery Room

OK, you've made it through. The operation is over, and you are as you've seen yourself all day—happy, healthy, and relaxed. (OK, maybe a little woozy, but hey, why not? You earned it.) You awaken wonderfully, perhaps with a slight ache or discomfort in the area of the surgery or a little sleepiness still from the medications, but you realize that like most things in life, it's the stress, anxiety, and anticipation that's generally the problem, not the actual event. And of course as with most operations, everything went according to plan, and all is well.

If by chance you are experiencing a few symptoms or side effects, here's what to do.

While you're in the recovery room let the nurses know that you're awake and feeling great. Hopefully they will ask you simply, "How do you feel?"

Tell them what you feel. If you feel great, super; that is wonderful, and frankly in many cases, exactly what we expect. Don't panic and think that unless you tell them that you're really

181

uncomfortable they won't give you anything. If you are uncomfortable, and your body needs something, your vital signs and blood pressure will tell that story.

Simply tell them how and what you feel—the good and the less happy, if it exists. They may offer you medicine or not. If you're just a bit uncomfortable, and generally this is about all you should be experiencing, count yourself back in and put yourself back in a relaxed state. Now remember, if you're not awake, they won't let you go home, but if they tell you that you will be there for a little while, enjoy the time; if they know you're using meditation and relaxation techniques, it's no big deal.

I had a family member who used self-hypnosis for surgery and of course, it went without a hitch. No discomfort, no problems, and when the surgeon came out to talk to me, he told me that recovery was going to be quite a bit of time because she was not waking up. I smiled and thanked him, and once he informed me that everything went great, I went back to visit her in the recovery room. I was told by the anesthesia people that they'd given minimal if any anesthetic and/or sedation at all. It should have worn off, but she didn't seem to be waking up. I smiled again and said OK. The recovery room nurse repeated the same litany to me and said, "You'll be here a while; you might as well go sit and relax."

I said, "Can I talk to her?"

She said, "Sure."

So I went in and said, "OK, the operation is over, and now it's time to count and wake yourself up so when we count from one to ten, you'll feel happy, healthy, wide awake and relaxed!"

This was the method we agreed upon for her to wake up after the procedure, so all I had to do was tell her all was good, and it was wake-up time. As soon as we hit ten, she jumped up, looked at the nurse, and said, "OK, I'm ready to go home." The nurse was startled and just shook her head in amazement.

I said, "Don't worry about it; this is hypnosis, and it really works!" We left fifteen minutes later and went out for Starbucks!

The key here is that you remain in control. You use medical meditation postoperatively just as you did in surgery. Use it to remind yourself you are happy, healthy, and relaxed, feeling great, and that your healing has already occurred. Use your little triggers to deal with any discomforts and anxieties that go along with your post-op sensations or feelings.

Remember you are in control; you're in charge. Be aware of things in your body, but don't be afraid of them. Your body's way of telling you that it's alive and still kicking is to have a little bit of discomfort or experience a little bit of a twinge in the area where it was worked on. This normal feeling or sensation is quite different from one that requires medication. If you need meds, you will know it. Generally speaking, with normal soreness, it's just your body telling you to be careful with this area and go a little easy. Once you look at things this way and reset your mental thermostat to understand that the discomfort is there to keep you from doing too much and to protect you, not to hurt you, you realize it's your friend. Befriend it and use it to your benefit. Don't be afraid of it; let it empower you.

What if I'm in the recovery room and I really feel uncomfortable?

This is what medicine is for. You haven't failed anything if you take medication. All you've done is realize that whatever is going on, it's slightly more than your mind wants to handle at that point and time—and that is perfectly fine. This is what you have prepared for, to be OK with or without postoperative medication. Remember that discomfort is your friend, and if it is a lot, it means that you should let your medical professionals know about it. But you will likely need a lot less medicine than you would have if you didn't use the medical meditation, which means this is safer, and you will also have less hangover effects from it.

So once again get in touch with what you're really feeling. If it's panic or anxiety, this is one thing. If on the other hand you're really hurting, just ask for something, and they will give you medication. The same goes with feeling a little dizzy or a little anxious post-op. Remember you are just waking up from a very, very deep nap. Let your body reorient and take your time. There is never a rush; just taking your time and letting your body naturally awaken and come to is the best way to go. Try to drink something when you wake up if you are allowed and continue to focus on your triggers and the image you've placed in your mind of you...happy, healthy, relaxed, done with your procedure, and already healed.

What if after the surgery I'm really just not feeling right, and I feel like I'm losing control?

We all panic and have doubts. This is normal. As silly as it sounds, just remember to breathe! Take a few deep breaths and let them out slowly. The key is to continue to use the techniques you have learned and also remember it is absolutely fine and appropriate to ask the medical staff for help.

As long as you continue to remind yourself that you control your mind and body, as well as see your happy image of you as healing already, happy and healthy, everything will continue just as planned. Most all of us falter at one time or another and doubt our own minds, whether it's with everyday decisions or meditation. We are all human, and weak moments are simply opportunities to regroup and the most important times to remind ourselves that we control our minds and bodies. So when we falter, the best answer is simply...do it more. Remember the four golden rules of how to take care of you; these are the keys to your success. Practice is the biggest thing. The more you do it and redo it and use it, especially when you think it's not working as well as you would like, the better it gets.

*For those suffering and facing daily challenges...*these techniques and the above advice not only apply to postoperative patients but to anyone who is facing the same challenges in dealing with daily life, be it stress, opioid dependence, or inability to sleep. The challenges are essentially the same: how to deal with suffering in the face of a situation where we are still raw from coming off a difficult experience. The advice and answers are all the same...go back to your breathing, let go of the anxiety and stress, breathe through the discomfort, and maintain control of your mind and body. You are in charge, and you alone have the ability to maintain that control and heal or feel better while you dictate when you need help or how much you can handle at any one time or on any given day. You may be surprised to learn how strong each one of us is when we believe in ourselves and our body's innate ability to care for itself. All we really need to do is give our subconscious mind permission to take care of us, and indeed that is exactly what it does!

Remember The Four Golden Rules

Rule Number 1: When you feel stressed, put yourself in.

Rule Number 2: Put yourself in whenever you want, not just when and because you think you should.

Rule Number 3: Take time every day for your medical meditation and self-hypnosis—happily guilt-free, enjoying and embracing the special time and gift you give yourself.

Rule Number 4: Don't miss a day!

CHAPTER 44

Your Grand Finale!

All of man's miseries derive from his inability to
sit quietly in a room alone.
—Blaise Pascal

How to Make It Work after You're Home

Remember that by doing medical meditation/self-hypnosis and imprinting an image in your subconscious mind of you as happy, healthy, and relaxed, you began your healing long before the incision is made, or you gave up the last pill you thought you couldn't live without. Your body began priming itself to have enhanced immune function, increased blood flow, and circulation to the area being treated or causing the most discomfort, and to be relaxed. Further, you began priming your mind and body for a post-op program or a life that did not depend on external medications to feel good or enjoy life to its fullest. Your personal healing, rehabilitation, and conditioning program began long before you took that car ride to the hospital or made a choice to take charge of your own healing. You already have the tools to teach yourself to relax, decrease discomfort, re-channel your thoughts, and to feel better—the key is to continue that habit and continue that conditioning. You now can begin to tailor your practice—instead of anticipating an anxious or uncomfortable day, you begin expecting wonderful days, every day. The same thoughts and practices that got you through your surgery so easily or to not take that extra pill now allow your body to heal and recuperate more quickly and effectively. Your body knows how to heal; it knows how to bring new cells to an area that needs repair, to form good, solid, soft, and pliable scar tissue and rid itself of infection or toxic invaders as well as revitalize your organs and tissues. The key to healing: I've told you this once, twice, or a thousand times, and is so simple it seems too good to be true...what you envision becomes your reality! So you choose how you look and feel as happy, healthy, and relaxed, your vision or picture—and it has no choice but to manifest. Your subconscious mind then sends exactly the right hormones to exactly the right areas of your body to bring about exactly the right response to achieve the healing and happiness you envision.

Medical meditation and self-hypnosis and the happy images in your subconscious mind never stop working for you. Your subconscious mind knows only to please you, so when you see yourself as happy, healthy, and relaxed that is exactly what it will create. All you really need do is continue to envision what you want and how you want it, and it will simply manifest.

If it sounds like I'm oversimplifying this, don't let it fool you. People have been healing, self-healing, comforting themselves and those they love, and achieving miracles through belief and focusing their thoughts for centuries. Be it self-hypnosis, meditation, religious prayer, faith healing, or laying on of hands, it is all the same. As long as you see it, know it will happen, and believe, it will occur exactly as you desire.

A few final thoughts:

You cannot isolate your mind from your body. Along with healing through medical meditation, relaxation, and visualizing yourself as healthy, there are two other vital aspects to the triad for long-term health and happiness. These are eating healthfully and a little exercise.

Let's talk food for a few minutes. To clarify I do not mean you need a strict or limited diet, one with a rigid fixed set of rules, but rather to simply modify, add, or subtract certain items to what you do or don't enjoy eating. Thankfully today, with access to so many different fresh foods, it is easier than ever. The key is finding balance.

Try to visualize your own ideal weight and how wonderfully healthy you feel when you are eating a reasonable diet. That vision is how you think you look best, not how the internet defines perfect! Too much in any one direction, any extreme, is usually not optimally healthy.

In general less red meat and less meat overall, as well as more fruits and a good balance of protein to carbohydrates in your diet, makes a world of difference. Ideally add more green or leafy vegetables, fish if it's to your taste, and stay away from fried or high-cholesterol foods. As to drinks, water is key to life, so get enough in you as well as limiting or even eliminating sugary drinks like soda and many of the sweetened teas and coffees. You don't need to be a purist; I must admit a great pleasure in occasional use of a sweetener in coffee or tea for one cup, although the rest of the day I enjoy a constantly refilled pot of green or white tea (decaffeinated for those who are caffeine sensitive). To decaffeinate any tea, just put in your tea leaves or a bag of tea and soak in hot water for a count of three. Then pour out that water and brew your tea. Caffeine is a very small molecule, and it easily comes out in the water. The good news is that the polyphenols and other healthy antioxidants in the tea are larger molecules so these along with the taste remain for you to enjoy.

Your body is primed this way to optimize its efficiency from the fuel that you give it and limits the oxidative damage that occurs from the foods that are bad for you. This is not to say you can't indulge in a cheeseburger or a little chocolate once in a while, but these should be treats, not the mainstay of your diet.

Concerning exercise, it is simply finding something that you like to let you move. Your body is an incredible machine, probably the most perfect machine we could conceive. It oils itself with lubrication, self-regulates, sweats when it overheats to cool down, and repairs its damaged parts. It eliminates toxins, allows us to interact with and adapt to all types of climates and situations, and it allows us to experience all the wonders of this world, from holding a newborn baby to the thrill of a roller coaster. All it asks of us is that we keep it moving so that it stays in condition to handle whatever the world throws at it. It enjoys moving and in fact feels better when it moves—your body, like any machine, gets stiff and begins to fall apart if it is not used regularly and taken care of.

Exercise can be as simple as standing at your desk instead of sitting all day, taking a walk, dancing, or even doing toning exercises while in bed or watching television. Exercises such as tai chi, Pilates, swimming, hiking, and yoga, any that keep the body moving but don't tear or repeatedly pound and deteriorate your joints are great. Some people who are lucky enough to have a job that also lets them stay active get double benefit from going to work.

The thing that is known about maintaining a level of activity in our lives is that moving the body enhances healing. The science is clear and has demonstrated that these activities allow the healing processes of the body to function better—producing lower blood pressure, lower cholesterol levels, decreased stress, and an extra plus, making you happy through the release of endorphins, enkephalins, and serotonin, the feel-good hormones. You don't need to go to the gym and sweat (but you can if you enjoy it), just move on a regular basis, be it walking, taking the stairs, or dancing. Find a form of exercise and movement and do it regularly. It will enhance your healing and your life.

And concerning healing postoperatively, the sooner you get moving, if your doctor says it's safe to do so, the better you'll do. Women used to stay in the hospital for a week after having babies; now they go home within a day or so—some don't even stay overnight at all. Not surprisingly, they have fewer complications and are generally happier mothers and children.

You now have all the tools to face this little challenge in your life. Buddha said, "It's all about suffering." What he meant is that there will always be challenges in life; in fact, that is what we are here for: to learn from, experience, and overcome these challenges and sufferings so that we emerge stronger and more resilient from each of them.

There will always be something that will test us or that we need to get through or get past, be it learning to walk, learning to write or ride a bicycle, or having a cold, a broken arm, or an operation. They're all basically the same. They're little challenges that tweak us in our life to become better. If you really think about it, all the things that you really feel good about, that you're proud of, that you have done or achieved, are those that you've had to work the hardest for and put extra effort into achieving. In fact the more the effort, and the more the challenge, the better you feel about it when you succeed. Life is not simply about having challenges and facing them, but even more so, embracing them. This doesn't mean going out and looking for trouble or an operation or a disease, but knowing that with the right attitude, a little preparation time and practice, you can handle anything!

I thank you, as I have so many of my patients over the years, for allowing me the privilege of sharing this journey with you. I look forward to hearing your stories and insights as well.

There are a few very special bonds you will form in your life if you're lucky: perhaps between you and your parents, siblings, significant other, child, trusted friend, clergy, or metaphysical, perhaps even mystical, friend.

The bond between you and your surgeon or doctor is a very special one. It is a trust where you give yourself, your actual being, completely over to them. You trust them literally with your life, your insides, and your survival. When you enter this kind of a relationship, you get to give something very special back. It is not just what they are doing for you but the nature of this bond is that you can do something for them – give your surgeon a sense and feeling of trust, love, and peace. They feel special thanks to your faith and this inexplicable bond. That peace you create through these techniques may well be an inner peace, but the radiance of that peace around you makes your doctor a better healer, and you heal better.

Card: The Four Golden Rules

Rule Number 1: When you feel stressed, put yourself in.

Rule Number 2: Put yourself in whenever you want, not just when and because you think you should.

Rule Number 3: Take time every day for your medical meditation and self-hypnosis—happily, guilt-free, and enjoying and embracing the special time and gift you give yourself.

Rule Number 4: Don't miss a day!

A card for your doctor:

Here is a card for you to give to your anesthesiologist, nurses, and doctor.

Hello, I am having surgery today, and I use medical medita-tion and relaxation to help with making this a calm and happy day—for me and for you as well.

Could you please help by doing the following:

- *Allow me to relax and rest as long as it is safe and not inconvenient for you or your team.*

- *Please do not mention the word "pain," but ask me simply, "How do you feel?" or "How are you doing?" instead. This helps me to focus on feeling great and to enhance the effectiveness of your medications.*

- *Please allow me to listen to my audio relaxation with my headphones before and if at all possible, during the procedure... and after. If you need to interrupt me to ask me something or for my safety, of course this is absolutely OK.*

- *Although I may appear asleep, I will be awake and aware enough to answer questions and do what you need me to do, and though I look like I am sleeping, I am really using medical meditation to relax.*

- *Lastly you and your team are very special. Thank you for indulging me and allowing me to help you to take care of me.*

MEDICAL DISCLAIMER

This book and any information contained within as well as the accompanying Audios are intended to be for general information purposes only. The content of any information is not intended to be medical advice, medical consultation or a substitute for medical advice from a qualified health care practitioner.

Any opinions expressed in this book are not meant to be relied upon as specific medical advice; rather, all information and opinions contained on this book are intended to be a guide to an understanding of general medical principles not specified to a particular person.

Persons viewing this book and listening to the audio are cautioned that care and treatment for any medical condition should only be undertaken after evaluation and authorization by a physician or other health care provider who can fully examine the condition, take a complete history and formulate a care plan with you. Although medical self-hypnosis is accepted as a part of treatment for many conditions, a complete medical evaluation is necessary to address concern and understanding of other treatments that may be indicated for your particular condition.

You should not use these techniques or listen to the audio portion of the program while driving, working with machinery or when doing any activity that requires concentration and attention.

Although the authors, editors and contributors have made every effort to ensure the accuracy and completeness of information contained on this book, it is difficult to ensure that all of the information is accurate, and the possibility of an error can never be entirely eliminated. The authors, editors and contributors disclaim any liability or responsibility for injury or damage to persons or property which is incurred as a consequence, directly or indirectly, of the use and application of any of the contents of this book as well as for any unintentional slights to any person or entity. It is the reader's responsibility to know and follow local care protocol as provided by the medical advisors directing their care. The editors, authors or contributors, nor any other party who has been involved in the preparation of or creation of this book warrant that the information contained herein is in every respect accurate or complete, and they are not responsible for any errors, omissions, inaccuracies, inconsistencies, misrepresentations or for the results obtained from the use of such information.

By reading and using the subject matter of this book and using the Audios, you agree that The Upper Extremity Institute, the Montgomery County Hand Center, Doctor in the House, Healing Books and its affiliates, including Dr. Scott Fried are not liable for any damages or claims you may have arising out of or in connection with this book.